HUMAN DIGNITY AND REPRODUCTIVE TECHNOLOGY

Edited by

Nicholas C. Lund-Molfese
Michael L. Kelly

University Press of America,® Inc.
Lanham · Boulder · New York · Toronto · Oxford

Copyright © 2003 by
University Press of America,® Inc.
4501 Forbes Boulevard
Suite 200
Lanham, Maryland 20706
UPA Acquisitions Department (301) 459-3366

PO Box 317
Oxford
OX2 9RU, UK

All rights reserved
Printed in the United States of America
British Library Cataloging in Publication Information Available

Library of Congress Control Number: 2003109236
ISBN 0-7618-2654-8 (paperback : alk. ppr.)

™
⊖ The paper used in this publication meets the minimum
requirements of American National Standard for Information
Sciences—Permanence of Paper for Printed Library Materials,
ANSI Z39.48—1984

CONTENTS

EDITOR'S NOTE

In March of 2002, the symposium *Human Dignity and Reproductive Technology* brought together a distinguished group of philosophers, theologians, scientists, lawyers, and scholars from across the United States. The Integritas Institute designed the symposium to examine the nature of human dignity in light of the tradition of the Catholic Church, and to relate this understanding to the proper application of modern reproductive technologies such as stem cell research, cloning, and in vitro fertilization.

As a necessary part of this project, the symposium implicitly recognized the complementary nature of both faith and reason. The Catholic faith proclaims the value and meaning of the human person in light of revelation, while reason (as science and philosophy) examines the human person in his physical dimensions. Considering the human person under both of these aspects is essential to the formation of law and public policy in accordance with human dignity.

The essays that appear in this book are the contribution of each of the symposium's participants. They have been organized into three sections that approach the topic from different perspectives. The first section describes the current cultural notions of human dignity and reproductive technology, the problems inherent in that understanding, and the work needed to remedy the loss of respect for human life in modern culture. The second section approaches human dignity and reproductive technology from a philosophical perspective. It attempts to assign a proper role to modern science and technology in order to preserve and protect the sanctity of human life. The third and final section describes the current political and legal context in which this debate is taking place.

It is our intention that in bringing together these essays, we present Catholic positions concerning human life and modern science. We hope to diagnose the fundamental moral defects of our culture in order to define the spiritual and intellectual work needed to preserve respect for the sanctity of human life and institutions such as marriage and the family. We would like to express our gratitude to Francis Cardinal George, the John Paul II Newman Center, and the Catholic Physician's Guild for their support.

INTRODUCTION

Patrick Guinan

The theme of the 2002 John Paul II Newman Center's Symposium "Human Dignity and Reproductive Technology" contrasts two ambiguous subjects that are potentially on a collision course. Ambiguous because "dignity" and "technology" are ascribed different meanings, and on a collision course because human dignity, as it should be understood, is incompatible with reproductive technology as it is currently being pursued.

We will first define human dignity and then explain how it is understood in our modern culture. Second, we will review the development of science and its stepchild technology, especially in the area of reproductive technology. Finally, we will note how human dignity, properly understood, restrains reproductive technology as that field is currently being developed.

Human Dignity

There are two traditions regarding the value of the human person. Modern culture, the product of the Enlightenment, defines the human person in terms of the rights that a person is entitled to. The more classical or Greco-Judeo-Christian philosophical tradition considers the person to have an inherent dignity because it is inherent in human nature and a corollary of the fact that man is made in the image of God. There is a fundamental difference between these traditions.

The Enlightenment can be considered the origin of our modern culture. In essence, it was a Pelegian effort promoting the perfectibility of man. For a variety of reasons, including Occam's nominalism, the classic Aristotelian realist tradition lost its teaching authority. In its place, a blend of Descartes' idealism, Locke's empiricism, and Hobbe's social contract resulted in a philosophy that understood humankind as warring savages who must bond together in order to surrender individual authority to the state, which in turn granted rights to its citizens. Rights were not inherent to the person but conferred. This trend continued through the nineteenth century with the development of liberal democracy in the United States and Great Britain.

Unfortunately, the totalitarianism of the twentieth century—particularly in Germany, the Soviet Union, and in many other countries—has put the lie to Enlightenment utopianism and its definition of rights. Millions have suffered and died in spite of state guaranteed rights. It should be noted that Hitler, in 1933, was democratically elected.

It is painfully evident that the state, given the Nazi and Communist models, cannot be the guarantor of human rights. Yet, ever more encompassing efforts are being made to do just that. Currently the United Nation's "Universal Declaration of Human Rights" is the instrument presumably guaranteeing all human rights. The document is significant in that unlike the United States Declaration of Independence, which acknowledges the divine origin of human rights, this document declares that human rights flow from a United Nation's declaration. Presumably, these rights could be changed or denied should that body decide to do so.

The second, or classical tradition of human dignity predates the Enlightenment. It is the Greco-Judeo-Christian tradition, which states that man is a rational animal consisting of an animating soul in a human body. Because the soul has an intellect and a will, it is immaterial and permanent. These attributes give it qualities not found in brute animals. In addition to the Greek concept, the Judeo-Christian tradition claims that man is made in the image of God and that Jesus Christ, the Son of God, became man to redeem mankind. This tradition places the origin of human dignity and rights in human nature itself and not in the state or organized government.

The classical and Enlightenment traditions of human dignity clash in many areas including law, the family, and education. Another area of conflict is in the application of technology, especially in the area of reproductive biology.

Reproductive Technology

Science, the ordered understanding of nature, can be considered to have originated in Aristotle's deductive observations about the natural world. Modern inductive science is attributed to Francis Bacon and Rene Descartes. It consists of hypotheses made from data collected from reproducible observations of physical events, and ultimately theories or models integrating these hypotheses to explain the natural world.[1]

The word technology is derived from the Greek word "techne" meaning art or craft. It is applied science, that is, it takes scientific theory and makes it practical or productive. Nuclear fission is science, whereas atomic power, whether it is a destructive atomic bomb or a nuclear reactor to produce electric power, is an example of technology.

Science is value neutral inasmuch as scientific knowledge is simply data, the collection and analysis of measurable events in nature. Technology has an ethical dimension because in its application it may do either good or harm. Nuclear energy may either be used for good, the production of electricity, or for evil, as an atomic explosion that kills innocent civilians.

Technology has been a mixed blessing. While universally acclaimed in the nineteenth and first half of the twentieth centuries, it has come under increasing scrutiny. Jacques Ellul, the French sociologist, was perhaps technology's most perceptive critic. His two concerns were: (1) Does the technological imperative determine social ends and (2) Can man remain free if he is hostage to technology?[2] These questions have ethical implications.

Reproductive technology is a case in point. It takes science, observations regarding human reproduction, and conducts experiments to achieve a desired result in the real world. Stem cell research and cloning are two examples. Stem cells are cells observed early in an organism's development. They have the potential to develop into a variety of more mature cell lines such as blood, digestive, or nerve cells. Stem cells can be obtained from a variety of sources such as cord blood, adipose tissue, or frozen embryos. Taking stem cells and stimulating them with growth factors to produce neural cells is one example of this technology.

Cloning, another reproductive technology, is the transfer of a full complement of forty-six human chromosomes from a somatic cell into an enucleated ovum, and then stimulating that cell to divide. The dividing cells can then be used for therapeutic or reproductive purposes.

It is evident that ethical considerations are at play regarding stem cells and cloning. Stem cells can be legitimately obtained from cord blood and adipose tissue. Destroying a human embryo, a human person, albeit at its earliest stage to obtain stem cells, is the deliberate killing of a human person and unethical. So also, cloning a human person artificially is immoral because human persons are ends in themselves and not to be used as means, which is the problem inherent in cloning technology. Moreover, cloning a person is in violation of God's plan for the generation of human life, which is the conjugal act of a husband and wife.

Aside from the specific issues of stem cells and cloning, there is the larger question of the possible limits on technology, as alluded to by Ellul, and even some aspects of the unrestrained pursuit of knowledge itself.[3]

Human Dignity Can Limit Technology

The classical tradition was God centered. While man was the most noble of creatures, he existed in the natural order and was subject to the rules of a finite and material existence. The modern Enlightenment order is man centered and as such views man in a Pelegian manner, that is, as limitless and perfectible. Man can know and do all things, hence the technological imperative.

The classical literary tradition reflects the acknowledged limits on what man can do and know, and the consequences for those who attempt to exceed these limits. For example, Icarus, given wings by Daedalus, wanted to fly closer to the sun than was allowed. This, however, was impossible and his wings melted with tragic results. Hubris, the Greek concept of tragic pride, is the human effort to do and know more than is the lot of man, and by implication, what is therefore forbidden by God. Adam and Eve ate the denied fruit and suffered the inevitable consequences. Man attempts to be equal to God, cannot, and is punished.

These themes are repeated in the more recent literature and scientific discoveries. Oppenheimer regretted making the atomic bomb, for example. In the literary world, Mary Shelly's Dr. Frankenstein wanted to create life. He made a monster that became a killer, and then regretted his actions. Faust signed a pact with Mephistopheles for knowledge and lost his soul. There is an acknowledgment in the literature that there are limits to human technical ability and dangers in the unrestrained pursuit of knowledge. At times, the scientific and academic communities do not seem to grasp this insight.

In summary, the Enlightenment project assumed a Pelegian posture. Man controls his destiny, is captain of his ship. While the tenets of modern science have been questioned in a postmodern critique by Thomas Kuhn,[4] scientific hubris and the technological imperative remain in the ascendancy.

In general, our larger society views human dignity from the Greco-Judeo-Christian perspective. It recognizes that embryos are persons that should not be destroyed for pragmatic purposes. It also rejects cloning as a Dr. Frankenstein form of monster creation. However, the Enlightenment-utilitarian approach would appear to be favored by many in the scientific establishment, the knowledge class, and the media. The fact that in contemporary liberal democracy, rights flow from the government either by legislation, or more recently by judicial fiat, tends to reinforce an imperative to pursue this research. Can man do as he pleases, or are there limits?

The human person has an innate dignity by his nature. This dignity precludes treating a person as a means, as would be the case in embryonic stem cell research and cloning. These two competing cultural forces are engaged in this important discussion, the subject of the 2002 John Paul II Newman Center's Symposium. The issues go beyond stem cells and cloning to what it means to be a person and how that person is to be protected.

As Cardinal George mentioned in his Opening Remarks we have the opportunity "to pursue the dialogue that will determine the place of human beings in a truly new world." Let us hope and pray that the dialogue of this Symposium will truly promote human dignity.

Notes

1. William Wallace, *Modeling of Nature* (Washington, DC: Catholic University of American Press, 1996).
2. Jacques Ellul, *The Technological Society* (New York, NY: Vintage Books, 1964).
3. Roger Shattuck, *Forbidden Knowledge* (San Diego, CA: Harcourt Branch and Co., 1996).
4. Thomas Kuhn, *The Structure of the Scientific Revolution* (Chicago, IL: The University of Chicago Press, 1962).

1

Part I:

Culture, Technology, and the Church

CHAPTER 1

Opening Remarks

Francis Cardinal George, O.M.I.

The topic "Human Dignity and Reproductive Technology" has great significance far beyond this gathering. The decisions made about the relationship between human dignity and reproductive technology, by individuals in pursuing their own goals and their self-understanding of who they are, form the public opinion, which influences governments, governmental agencies, and non-governmental economic organizations as well. All these decisions collectively shape the new global order that is coming into being.

Cumulatively, these decisions will determine the place of human beings in a truly New World. Economic and political dynamisms that are shaping a global society have their own internal laws, and we are more familiar with how those work themselves out in public then we are with the technological dynamism that is involved in the advance of the biological sciences.

It is our hope in sponsoring a conference such as this, and in your coming together to be a part of the symposium, that principles of morality, principles that are faith-based in part but are also open to discussion by all people of good will, will be articulated and argued. These principles must enter into the dynamics of technology as implemented by political entities and economic agencies in order to uphold human dignity and to humanize whatever world culture or world order we are moving towards.

In this new context in which a truly global civilization struggles to be born, there should be considerable philosophical and moral discussion. We are here in a seminar sponsored by Catholic intellectuals and Catholic agencies, professionals in their own fields, and hopeful, therefore, of being able to bring their faith and their professions into productive dialogue. But, if there is to be an impact, then we need great clarity about the scientific goals and the technological procedures. We need also a deepened of understanding of exactly how our principles, derived from faith, might lead us to take part in this conversation. And we need a certain moral stamina or courage in order to sustain that conversation even when the outcome is uncertain or when in fact there is considerable opposition to our own positions. All of these goals are in some sense within the scope of this symposium, and I am extremely grateful that it is taking place.

There are fundamental, intrinsic goods, if you like, that everyone holds whether thematically, self-consciously, or not. Faith keeps coming back to human dignity because human beings are made in God's image and likeness. The scientific community keeps talking about an advance in human knowledge and therefore in our capacity to understand and use nature in such a way that physical nature serves human purposes. These are intrinsic goods, goods in themselves, and they need to be respected. Where they seem to clash is the point of discussion in this and in many similar symposia and conferences.

I am grateful that we have the opportunity to pursue that conversation today, grateful to the speakers, and grateful to those who have organized such a truly outstanding roster of speakers. I am especially grateful to those in the Integritas Institute who have sponsored this, Nicholas Lund-Molfese and Kara Alden, who have worked also with Fr. Pat Marshall of the John Paul II Newman Center and his staff in order to make this conference a much desired and hoped for reality. Finally, I would like to express a note of deep gratitude to Chancellor Sylvia Manning for leading a university open to such dialogue, and therefore a place of genuine learning that brings hope of progress for us all. Thank you very much.

CHAPTER 2

The Body and the Quest for Control

Jean Bethke Elshtain

In our fast-paced, fitness and youth oriented culture, perfecting the human body has become a messianic project. In this essay, I bring theological anthropology to bear on this project for the purpose of critique. It is not that easy, of course, to stand apart from the dominant preoccupations of one's own culture in order to assess its enthusiasms critically. But, I take this to be an essential task, difficulties notwithstanding.

The situation that we face is this: bodies are thought of increasingly as the exclusive property of an individual for him or her to do with as he or she sees fit. Bodies are also construed as malleable and 'constructable.' We are all enjoined, through advertising, cultural imagery on television and in films, science joined to profit in the bio-tech industry, popularizers of the genetic revolution, and others, to "get with the program," to hop on board and not remain stuck in superstition that urges restraint or even curtailment of genetic and biological engineering.

Philosophers and cultural critics indebted to Christianity, among whom I number myself, are poised as a matter of principle and faithfulness in a tension between *contra mundum* and *amor mundi* in ways that may be fruitful, frustrating, or both. This tension begins with the recognition that uncritical identification with the currents of one's own time is easily understood because so many of those currents speak to real human needs, fears, desires, and the goods associated with these. Therein lies a major part of the problem, at least if one follows Martin Luther's lead. Luther insisted that all our needs are bound to be distorted given human rebellion against God, beginning with that Ur-disobedience that got Adam and Eve thrown out of the Garden. Ever since, the human being is marked by a trace of this original willfulness, or so argued the great reformer. We are separated from God, the source of undistorted love. In addition, given that Christian theological anthropology presumes intrinsic relationality—there is no primordial free self—sifting our cherished and essential commonalties (and communealities) from unthinking absorption in dominant cultural forces is bound to be a delicate matter.

As the essay proceeds, I will take up examples of cultural acquiescence in ever-more radical manipulations of the human body.[1] An overarching and framing thematic of contemporary American culture is a flight from finitude that undermines recognition of the complexities and limits as well as the joys of embodiment—the givens, if you will, of human *being* itself. One spin-off is widespread approval in the destruction of the bodies of others as part of our culture's panoply of invented rights and punishments, whether *in situ* (the abortion regime) or as a central feature of our system of retributive justice (the death penalty.)[2] Neither the abortion "right" nor capital punishment is a focus of this essay, but insofar as each practice involves the destruction of a human body, one developing and the other developed, these practices help to structure the overall cultural frame concerning the differential value we assign to some human bodies in contrast to others.

Having noted Luther's mordant view of the lingering implications of human defiance of the Creator, let's flesh matters out, beginning with reminders about the nature of Christian freedom and the fact that we are both creatures and creators. As creatures we are dependent. It follows that our creaturely freedom consists in our recognition that we are not abstractly free but free only in and through relationship. A limit lies at the very heart of our existence in freedom. Christian freedom turns on recognition of the limits to freedom.

German theologian and anti-Nazi martyr, Dietrich Bonhoeffer, in *Creation and Fall*, frets that man as creator easily transmogrifies into a destroyer as he or she misuses freedom.[3] There is a big difference between enacting human projects as co-creators respectful of a limit because, unlike God, we are neither infinite nor omniscient and, by contrast, enacting those projects that demand that humans embrace God-likeness for themselves, up to the point of displacing God Himself. With God removed as a brake on human self-sovereignty, we see no limit to what human power might accomplish. An alternative to this project of self-overcoming is an understanding of a humbler freedom, a freedom that never aspires to the absolute. This freedom is constitutive of our natures. Theologian Robin Lovin helps us to appreciate a specifically Christian freedom that is not opposed to the natural order but acts in complex faithfulness to it.[4]

One begins by taking human beings as they are, not as those fanciful entities sometimes conjured up by philosophers in what they themselves call "science fiction" examples.[5] To be sure, the freedom of a real, not a fanciful, human being means, among other things, that one can "project oneself imaginatively into a situation in which the constraints of present experience no longer hold."[6] One can imagine states of perfection or nigh-perfection. At the same time, actual freedom is always situated; it is not an abstract position located nowhere-in-particular. Freedom is concrete, not free-floating. Freedom is a "basic human good. Life without freedom is not something we would choose, no matter how comfortable the material circumstances might be."[7] Our reasoning capacity is part and parcel of our freedom. But, that reasoning is not a separate faculty cut off from our embodied selves; instead it is profoundly constituted by our embodied histories and memories.

Christian freedom, in Lovin's words, consists in our ability to "avoid excessive identification with the surrounding culture, since that tends both to lower...moral expectations and to deprive [persons] of the witness to alternative possibilities...."[8] If the horizon lowers excessively, the possibility that we might exercise our capacity for freedom is correlatively negated. So the denial of freedom consists, in part, in a refusal to accept the freedom that is the human inheritance of finite, limited creatures "whose capacities for change are also limited, and who can only bring about new situations that are also themselves particular, local, and contingent."[9] To presume more than this is also problematic, launching us into dangerous hubris often, of course, in the name of great ideals, like choice or justice. So our freedom is, at one and the same time, both real and limited.

With this as a backdrop, let's examine several contemporary projects of self-overcoming that involve a negation (or an attempt to negate) finitude and that rely on an uncritical endorsement of dominant cultural demands.[10] Such projects, remember, are tricky to approach critically because they present themselves to us in the dominant language of our culture—choice, consent, control—and promise an escape from the vagaries of the human condition into a realm of near mastery. Consider the fact that we are in the throes of a culture of biological obsession underwritten by pictures of absolute self-possession.[11] We are bombarded daily with the promise that nearly every human ailment or condition can be overcome if we just have sufficient will and skill, and refuse to listen to any entreaties from critics, who are invariably portrayed as negative and anti-progress. For those, philosopher Charles Taylor calls the "cultural boosters," our imperfect embodiment is a problem that must be overcome. For example, a premise—and promise—driving the Human Genome Project, the massive mapping of the genetic code of the entire human race, is that we might one day intervene decisively in order to guarantee better if not perfect human products.[12] Claims made by promoters and advocates of this project run to the ecstatic.

Take, for example, Walter Gilbert's 1986 pronouncement that "[The Humane Genome Project] is the grail of human genetics...the ultimate answer to the commandment, 'Know thyself.'"[13] In the genome-enthusiast camp, they are already talking about Designer Genes. Note, in this regard, the following advertisement reported by *The New York Times* in early Spring, 1999, an ad that had appeared in college newspapers all over the country: "EGG DONOR NEEDED/LARGE FINANCIAL INCENTIVE/INTEL-LIGENT, ATHLETIC EGG DONOR NEEDED/FOR LOVING FAMILY/ YOU MUST BE AT LEAST 5'10"/ HAVE A 1400+ SAT SCORE/POS-SESS NO MAJOR FAMILY MEDICAL ISSUES/$50,000/ FREE MEDICAL SCREENING/ALL EXPENSES PAID."[14] As *Commonweal* noted in an editorial occasioned by this advertisement, this brings back eerie reminders of earlier advertisements that involved trade in human flesh (the reference point being the slave trade) and suggests that "we are fast returning to a world where persons carry a price tag, and where the cash value of some persons...is far greater than that of others."[15]

More sober voices, like that of scientist Doris T. Zallen, find themselves struggling to gain a hearing above the din of enthusiastic rhetoric. Having noted that the early promises of genetic intervention to forestall "serious health problems, such as sickle-cell anemia, cystic fibrosis, and Huntington disease," have thus far had only the most meager success, Zallen takes up this booming genetic enterprise that promises not prevention of harm, but the attainment of perfection. It is called "genetic enhancement." One starts with a healthy person and then moves to perfect. Zallen calls this the "genetic equivalent of cosmetic surgery." The aim is to make people "taller, thinner, more athletic, or more attractive." Zallen lists potential harms, including reinforcement of "irrational societal prejudices. For instance, what would happen to short people if genetic enhancement were available to increase one's height?" The "historical record is not encouraging," she adds, noting the earlier eugenics movement and its hideous outcomes, most frighteningly in Nazi Germany, but evident in this country as well where policies of involuntary sterilization of persons with mental retardation and other measures went forward apace.[16]

The calmer voices remind us that the scientific community at present has only the "vaguest understanding" of the details of genetic instruction—unsurprising when one considers that each "single-celled conceptus immediately after fertilization [sic] involves a l00-trillion-times miniaturized information system..."[17] Yet, the enthusiasts who claim that the benefits of genetic manipulation are both unstoppable and entirely beneficial, downplay any and all controversies and short-circuit any and all difficulties. In this way, they undercut (or attempt to) any and all "non-expert" criticism in a manner that "effectively precludes others coming to an independent judgment about the validity of their claims."[18] The upshot is that it is very difficult to have the ethical and cultural discussion we require. Those who try to promote such are tagged with the label of "technophobes" or "Luddites."

Despite this, there are a few critical straws in the cultural wind. In the 1997 film, "Gattaca," for example, the protagonist (played by Ethan Hawke) is born the "old-fashioned way" (a "faith-birth") to his parents who had made love and taken their chances with what sort of offspring might eventuate. In this terrible new world, when a child is born an immediate genetic profile is done. Our protagonist, Vincent, is a beautiful but, it turns out, genetically hapless child (on the standards of the barren world that is to be his lot). He enters life, not amidst awe and hopefulness, but misery and worry. His mother clutches the tiny newborn to her breast as his genetic quotient is coldly read-off by the expert. "Cells tell all," the prophets of genoism intone. Because of his genetic flaws, for his was an unregulated birth, young Vincent isn't covered by insurance; he doesn't get to go to school past a certain age; and he is doomed to menial service. He is a degenerate. Or, as the scanners immediately pronounce it, an "Invalid."

Vincent contrives a way to fake-out the system as he yearns to go on a one-year manned mission to some truly far-out planet. Only "Valids"—genetically correct human beings—are eligible for such elite tasks. So Vincent pays off a "Valid" for the valid's urine, blood, saliva, and fingerprints and begins his arduous, elaborate ruse. For this is a world in which any bodily scraping—a single eyelash, a single bit of skin sloughing—might betray you. Why would a valid sell his bodily fluids and properties? Because the valid is now "useless," a cripple, having been paralyzed in a car accident. Indeed, his life is so useless on society's standards that he, in turn, has thoroughly internalized that, and after having stored sufficient urine and blood so that Vincent can fool the system for years to come, the crippled valid manages to ease himself into a blazing furnace, life not worth living any longer, at least not for one who cannot use his legs.

As for Vincent, and despite some very tense moments, life is as good as it is ever going to get by the film's end. He has made love to Uma Thurman and he has faked his way (with the connivance of a sympathetic security officer) onto the mission to the really far-out planet of which he has dreamt since childhood, despite his genetically flawed condition. This is a bleak film. The only resistance Vincent can come up with is faking it. He has no language of protest and ethical distance available to him. This is just the world as he and others know it and presumably will always know it. Uma Thurman's intimacy with an Invalid is as close to resistance as she can get.[19] There are no alternative points of reference or resistance.

Of course, we are not in the "Gattaca" nightmare yet. But are we drawing uncomfortably close? There are those who believe so, including the mother of a Down syndrome child who wrote me after she had read one of my columns about genetic engineering in *The New Republic*. In that piece, I reflected on what our quest for bodily perfection might mean over the long run for the developmentally different. My interlocutor, whose child died of a critical illness in his third year, wrote me that she and her husband were enormously grateful to have had "the joyous privilege of parenting a child with Down syndrome...Tommy's [not his real name] birth truly transformed our lives in ways that we will cherish forever. But, how could we have known in advance that we indeed possessed the fortitude to parent a child with special needs? And who would have told us of the rich rewards?" She continued:

> The function of prenatal tests, despite protestations to the contrary, is to provide parents the information necessary to assure that all pregnancies brought to term are 'normal'. I worry not only about the encouragement given to eliminating a 'whole category of persons' (the point you make), but also about the prospects for respect and treatment of children who come to be brain-damaged either through unexpected birth traumas or later accidents. And what about the pressures to which parents like myself will be subject? How could you 'choose' to burden society in this way?

In the name of expanding choice, we are narrowing our definition of humanity and, along the way, a felt responsibility to create welcoming environments for all children. If we simply declare that,—"they chose to have an 'abnormal' child and now they must pay the consequences," then this declaration, if it is generalized, takes us as individuals and a society off the hook for the purpose of social care and concern for all persons, including those with bodies and minds that are not "normal." The trend stitches together a cluster of views under the rubric of expanding choice, enhancing control, and extending freedom. The end result is diminution of the sphere of the "unchosen" and expansion of the reign of "control-over." Rather than viewing children who are not developmentally "normal" simply as a type of child who occurs from time-to-time among us and who, in common with all children, makes a claim on our most tender affections and most fundamental obligations, we see such children as beset by a "fixable" condition." We focus solely on the cure. The cure, for the most part, is to gain sufficient knowledge (or at least to claim to have such knowledge) that one can predict the outcome of a pregnancy and move immediately to prevent a "wrongful" birth in the first place. The fact that "curing" Down Syndrome means one eliminates entirely a type of human being is no barrier to this effort. People alive with Down Syndrome must simply live with the knowledge that our culture's dominant view is that it would be better if no more of their "kind" were to appear among us.

In a recent book, *The Future of the Disabled in Liberal Society: An Ethical Analysis*, philosopher Hans S. Reinders argues that, despite public policy efforts to ensure equal opportunity and access for all, liberal society (including our own) cannot sustain equal regard for persons with disabilities. This is especially true if the disabilities in question are "mental." The liberal presupposition which privileges "choice" as the primary concern in public life and the apogee of human aspiration, paired with modern technologies of reproductive and genetic engineering, dictate that it would be far better if human persons who are incapable of choosing on the liberal model were not to appear among us.

So strong is the prejudice in this direction that we simply assume that hypothetical unborn children with cognitive disabilities would, if they could, choose not to be born. Reinders, a professor of ethics at the Vrije University in Amsterdam, argues that the regnant view among liberal philosophers is that human beings with mental retardation may be regarded as members of the human species but they do not have full moral standing in the secular community.[20] Because they lack such standing, the barriers to eliminating such persons will slowly but surely wither away. To be sure, given the religious derivation of so much of our ethical thinking, barriers to simply killing persons with disabilities remain. But such barriers, Reinders argues, are under continuous pressure from "secular morality" and are likely to be bulldozed out of the way by the potent machine of biotechnology backed up by medical authority. So, it is not at all irrational for those with mental disabilities and their families to worry about the future. The proliferation of genetic testing, Reinders concludes, will most certainly have discriminatory effects because it puts everything under the domain of "choice," and parents of children with "special needs" become guilty of irresponsible behavior in "choosing" to bear such children and in burdening society in this way.

Increasingly, we as a society expect, and even insist, that parents must—for this is the direction "choice" takes at present—rid themselves of "wrongful life" in order to forestall "wrongful births" which will burden them, and even more importantly the wider society. Women repeatedly tell stories of the pressure from their medical caregivers to abort should a sonogram show up something suspicious. The current abortion regime often presents pregnancy as a burden for women who are told that they alone have the power to choose whether or not to have a child and that they alone are expected to bear the consequences if they do not choose to do so. The growing conviction that children with disabilities ought never to be born and that the prospective parents of such children ought always to abort undermines the felt skein of care and responsibility for all children.[21]

This is, at least, a reasonable worry especially when the machinery of technology now surrounding childbirth turns every pregnancy into what was once called a "crisis pregnancy." HMOs are now standardizing prenatal testing and genetic screening procedures, which were once called upon only when couples had a history of difficulties. The point of all this is to initiate a process—should a sign even be hinted at—"of cajoling and pressuring that terminates in an abortion...."[22] Jeannie Hannemann, a family life minister, "sees a culture shift taking place moving away from supporting families with special-needs children toward resenting such families as creating a 'burden' on society. [She] has heard of HMOs refusing treatment to special needs children, arguing their mental or physical problem represented a 'preexisting condition' because their parents elected not to abort them after prenatal screening indicated a problem."[23]

The heart of the matter lies in a loss of appreciation for the complex nature of human embodiment. The social imaginary—which the dominant scientific voices in the area of genetic engineering, technology, and "enhancement" shape—declares the body to be a construction, something we can invent. We are loathe to grant the status of "givenness" to any aspect of ourselves, despite the fact that human babies are wriggling, complex, little bodies pre-programmed with all sorts of delicately calibrated reactions to the human relationships that "nature" presumes will be the matrix of child nurture. If we think of bodies concretely in this way, we are propelled to ask ourselves questions about the world little human bodies enter. Is it welcoming, warm, and responsive? But, if we tilt in the bio-tech constructivist direction, one in which the body is so much raw material to be worked upon and worked over, the surrounding in which bodies are situated fades as "The Body" gets enshrined as a kind of messianic project.

In this latter scenario, the body we currently inhabit becomes the **imperfect body** subject to chance and the vagaries of life, including illness and aging. This body is our foe. The **future perfect body** extolled in manifestos, promised by enthusiasts, embraced by many ordinary citizens—is a gleaming fabrication. For soon, we are promised, we will have found a way around the fact that what our foremothers and forefathers took for granted— that the body must weaken and falter and one day pass from life to death—will soon be a relic of a by-gone era. The **future perfect body** will not be permitted to falter. Yes, the body may grow older in a strictly chronological sense, but why should we age? So we devise multiple strategies to fend off aging even as we represent aging bodies as those of teen-agers with gleaming gray hair. A recent *New York Times Magazine* lead article on "The Recycled Generation" extolled the "promise of an endless supply of new body parts" via stem cell research, although that research is now "bogged down in abortion politics and corporate rivalries."[24] One of the entrepreneurs who stands to make even more millions of dollars in what the article calls the "scientific chase" for "the mother of all cells—the embryonic stem cell"—bemoans the fact that the rush forward is being slowed down by a terrible problem, namely, the "knee jerk reaction" on the part of many people to "words like 'fetal' and 'embryo.'"

The image that came bounding out of the piece is that genetic innovators who face opposition from religious and superstitious people, who go "completely irrational" when they hear certain words, fearlessly forge forth in the teeth of sustained opposition. This, in fact, is a reversal of the actual situation in which critics are compelled to fight a rear-guard battle against a powerful, moneyed, and influential set of cultural forces that, in line with the story our culture likes to tell about itself, represent "progress" and a better future.[25] The outcome is that rather than approaching matters of life, death, and health with humility, knowing that we cannot cure the human condition, we seek cures in the assumption that the more we control the better. As I completed a final revision on this essay, word came that a human embryo had been cloned. Television commentary resounded with the promise that this will make possible, in the future, an endless supply of body parts that can be harvested to indefinitely prolong human life. Thus, even before a grown clone appears—and let us pray this does not happen—the clone is reduced to property to be harvested for the benefit of others.

The underlying presupposition is, of course, that nothing is good in itself, including embodied existence. Thus, it becomes easier to be rather casual about devising and implementing strategies aimed at selective weeding out or destruction of the "imperfect" or abnormal bodies, or even the bodies of the "perfect" if that human entity is cloned. Questions about whether the path we are racing down might not turn old age itself into a pathology, prompting cultural "encouragement" for the "unproductive" elderly to permit themselves to be euthanized, are cast aside as part of a science fiction dystopian mentality.

It is difficult to overstate just how widely accepted the technocratic view is and how overwhelmingly we, as a culture, acquiesce to its premises. In a review in the *Times Literary Supplement* of four new books on the genetic revolution, the reviewer matter-of-factly opined that "we must inevitably start to choose our descendants," adding that we do this now in "permitting or preventing the birth of our own children according to their medical prognosis, thus selecting the lives to come." So long as society does not cramp our freedom of action, we will stay on the road of progress and exercise sovereign choice over birth by consigning to death those with a less than stellar potential for a life not "marred by an excess of pain or disability."[26] Molecular biologist, Robert Sinsheimer, calls for a "new eugenics," a word most try to avoid given its association with the bio-political ideology of mid-twentieth century National Socialism. Sinsheimer writes, "The new eugenics would permit in principle the conversion of all the unfit to the highest genetic level."[27] In widespread adoption of prenatal screening, now regarded as routine so much so that prospective parents who decline this panoply of procedures are treated as irresponsible, we see at work the presumption that life should be wiped clean of any and all imperfection, inconvenience, and risk. Creation itself must be put right.

The New York Times, December 2, 1997, alerted us to this fact in an essay, "On Cloning Humans, 'Never' Turns Swiftly into 'Why Not'" by their science editor, Gina Kolata.[28] Kolata points out that in the immediate aftermath of Dolly, the cloned sheep who stared out at us from the covers of so many newspapers and magazines, there was much consternation and rumbling.[29] But, opposition dissipated quickly, she continues, with fertility centers soon conducting "experiments with human eggs that lay the groundwork for cloning. Moreover, the Federal Government is supporting new research on the cloning of monkeys, encouraging scientists to perfect techniques that could easily be transferred to humans." A Presidential ethics commission may have recommended a "limited ban on cloning humans,," but after all, "it is an American tradition to allow people the freedom to reproduce in any way they like." This claim is simply false to the historic and legal record. In common with any society of which we have any knowledge, past or present, American society has built into its interstices a variety of limitations on "reproductive freedom." But, the view that "freedom" means doing things in "any way one likes" now prevails as a cultural *desideratum*.[30] It is, therefore, unsurprising that *The New York Times* describes a "slow acceptance" of the idea of cloning in the scientific community that took but six months to go from shock and queasiness to acquiescence and widespread approval. The article concludes that, "some experts said the real question was not whether cloning is ethical but whether it is legal." And one doctor is quoted in these words, "The fact is that, in America, cloning may be bad but telling people how they should reproduce is worse.... In the end...America is not ruled by ethics. It is ruled by law." The implication of this view is that no ethical norm, standard, commitment, or insight can or should be brought to bear whether to criticize, to caution against, or to checkmate statutory laws should they be unjust or unwise. The point is that with each new development that is presented to us in the name of a radical and benign extension of human freedom and powers, we pave additional miles on the fast track toward eradication of any real integrity to the category of 'the human'. Debate and discourse about such matters in the public square has turned into a routine in which a few religious spokesmen or women are brought on board to fret a bit and everything marches on.[31]

The prospect that human cloning is fueled by narcissistic fantasies of radical sameness; that it represents fear of the different and the unpredictable; that it speaks for a world of guaranteed self-replication, matters not. Indeed, such concerns are rarely named save by those speaking from the point of view of theological anthropology. As The Pontifical Academy noted in a statement on human cloning issued June 25, 1997:

Human cloning belongs to the eugenics project and is thus subject to all the ethical and juridical observations that have amply condemned it. As Hans Jonas has already written, it is 'both in method the most despotic and in aim the most slavish form of genetic manipulation; its objective is not an arbitrary modification of the hereditary material but precisely its equally arbitrary fixation in contrast to the dominant strategy of nature.[32]

Dreams of strong, wholesale self-possession grounded in attaining full control over human "reproductive material" lie at the heart of the eugenics project. This carries the inherent risk of damaging biogenetic uniformity, since much of the basic genetic information that goes into the creation of a child from two parents emerges as a result of sexual reproduction, something not replicable by definition when you pick one parent to clone. The latter is evidently a small price to pay.

What, then, about embarking on an experimental course that would likely result in flawed "products?"[33] It is convenient to forget that it took nearly three hundred failed attempts before Dolly the sheep was cloned successfully. As Dr. Leon Kass has noted, the image of failed human clones leads the soul to shudder. Abandoning what Kass calls "the wisdom of repugnance," we embark on a path that constitutes a violation of a very fundamental sort. Kass calls upon us to pay close attention to what we find "offensive," "repulsive," or "distasteful," for such reactions often point to deeper realities. He writes, "...in this age in which everything is held to be permissible so long as it is freely done, in which our given human nature no longer commands respect, in which our bodies are regarded as mere instruments of our autonomous rational wills, repugnance may be the only voice left that speaks up to defend the central core of our humanity. Shallow are the souls that have forgotten how to shudder."[34] Kass is not arguing that repugnance is the end of the matter, but instead a beginning. Those philosophies that see in such reactions only the churning of irrational emotion, misunderstand the nature of human emotions. Our emotional reactions are complex, laced through and through with thought. The point is to bring forward such reactions and submit them to thought.

Would we really want to live in a world in which the sight of anonymous corpses piled up elicited no strong revulsion? A world in which the sight of a human being's body pierced through and through in dozens of places and riddled with pieces of metal was something we simply took for granted? The reaction to the first clearly gestures toward a powerful condemnation of those responsible for creating those mountains of corpses, and anguish and pity for the tortured and murdered and their families. In the case of the heavy-metal pierced person, we may decide it is a matter of little import and yet ask ourselves why mutilation of the body that goes much beyond the decorative is now so popular? Does this tell us anything about how we think about our bodies?[35]

Kass points out that the "technical, liberal, and meliorist approaches all ignore the deeper anthropological, social, and indeed, ontological meanings of bringing forth new life. To this more fitting and profound point of view, cloning shows itself to be a major alteration, indeed, a major violation, of our given nature as embodied, gendered, and engendering beings, and of the social relations built on this natural ground."[36] The upshot is that critical interpreters cede the ground too readily to those who want to move full steam ahead when, in fact, it should work the other way around. "The burden of moral argument must fall entirely on those who want to declare the widespread repugnancies of humankind to be mere timidity or superstition."[37] Too many theologians, philosophers, and cultural critics have become reticent about defending insights drawn from the riches of Western tradition.

As a result, Kass argues, we do the following things: we enter a world in which unethical experiments "upon the resulting child-to-be" are conducted; we deprive a cloned entity of a "distinctive identity not only because he will be in genotype and appearance to another human being, but, in this case, because he may also be twin to the person who is his 'father' or 'mother'—if one can still call them that"; we deliberately plan situations that we know—the empirical evidence is incontrovertible—are not optimal arenas for the rearing of children, namely, family fragments that deny relationality or shrink it; and we "enshrine and aggravate a profound and mischievous misunderstanding of the meaning of having children and of the parent-child relationship...The child is given a genotype that has already lived....Cloning is inherently despotic, for it seeks to make one's children...after one's own image...and their future according to one's will."[38] The many warnings imbedded in Western tradition, from its antique forms (pre-Christian) through Judaism and Christianity, seem now to lack the power to stay the hand of a 'scientized' anthropocentrism that distorts the meaning of human freedom.[39]

Within the Hebrew and Christian traditions, a burden borne by human beings after the fall lies in discerning what is natural or given. This, of course, presumes that that which is encoded into the very nature of things affords a standard, accessible to human reason by which we can critically assess the claims and forces at work in our cultural time and place. (This isn't the only available standard, of course, but it was long believed an important feature of a whole complex of views). The great moral teachers, until relatively recently, believed that "nature" and "the natural" served as a standard. Within Christian theological anthropology, human beings are corporeal beings, ensouled bodies, made in the image of their Creator. According to Pope John Paul II, this account of our natures, including the ontological equality of male and female as corporeal beings, is "free from any trace whatsoever of subjectivism. It contains only the objective facts and defines the objective reality, both when it speaks of man's creation, male and female, in the image of God, and when it adds a little later the words of the first blessing: 'Be fruitful and multiply and fill the earth; subdue it and have dominion over it'" (Gen. 1:28).[40] Dominion here—it is clear from the overall exegesis—is understood as a form of stewardship, not domination. John Paul's account of Genesis is presaged in Karol Wojtyla's prepapal writings. For example, in a series of spiritual exercises presented to Pope Paul VI, the papal household, and the cardinals and bishops of the Roman Curia during a Lenten Retreat in March 1976, then Cardinal Karol Wojtyla argued that "one cannot understand either Sartre or Marx without having first read and pondered very deeply the first three chapters of Genesis. These are the key to understanding the world of today, both its roots and its extremely radical—and therefore dramatic—affirmations and denials."[41] Teaching about human origins in this way offers "an articulation of the way things are by virtue of the relation they have with their creator."[42] Denying that relationship, we too easily fall into subjectivism, into a world of rootless wills.

With this Dietrich Bonhoeffer would agree. In his discussion of "The Natural" in the *Ethics*, Bonhoeffer observes that "the natural" fell out of favor in Protestant ethics and became the almost exclusive preserve of Catholic thought. He aimed to resurrect "the natural," insisting that human beings still have access to the natural but only "on the basis of the gospel."[43] In his move to redeem the concept of the natural, Bonhoeffer argues that human beings enjoy a "relative freedom" in natural life. But, there are "true and…mistaken uses of this freedom" and these mark "the difference between the natural and the unnatural." It follows that, "Destruction of the natural means destruction of life…The unnatural is the enemy of life."

It violates our natures to approach life from a false "vitalism" or excessive idealism, on the one hand, or on the other from an equally false "mechanization" and lassitude that shows "despair towards natural life" and manifests "a certain hostility to life, tiredness of life and incapacity for life." Our right to bodily life is a natural, not an invented right, and the basis of all other rights given that Christians repudiate the view that the body is simply a prison for the immortal soul. Harming the body harms the self at its depth. "Bodilyness and human life belong inseparably together," in Bonhoeffer's words. Our bodies are ends in themselves. This has "very far-reaching consequences for the Christian appraisal of all the problems that have to do with the life of the body, housing, food, clothing, recreation, play and sex." We can use our bodies and the bodies of others well or ill.

The most striking and radical excision of the integrity and right of natural life is "arbitrary killing," the deliberate destruction of "innocent life." Bonhoeffer notes abortion, killing defenseless prisoners or wounded men, and destroying lives we do not find worth living—a clear reference to Nazi euthanasia and genocidal policies toward the ill, the infirm, all persons with handicaps.[44] "The right to live is a matter of the essence" and not of any socially imposed or constructed values. Even "the most wretched life" is "worth living before God." Other violations of the liberty of the body include physical torture, arbitrary seizure and enslavement (American slavery is here referenced), deportations, and separation of persons from home and family—the full panoply of horrors the twentieth century has dished up in superabundance.

The fragment by Bonhoeffer on the natural is powerfully suggestive and worth pondering as an alternative to those cultural dictates that declare any appeal to nature or the natural as an illegitimate standard. It goes without saying that much more work would need to be done in order to redeem the categories of "nature" and "the natural." But, I want to simply note here that our present circumstances resist the possibility of this conceptual and ethical possibility, even as the need for some such standard becomes ever more exigent. We need powerful and coherent categories and analysis that challenge cultural projects that deny finitude and promise a technocratic agenda, which ushers in a future of almost total human control over all of the natural world, including those natures we call human. These cultural forces push us towards an ideal of sameness through genetic manipulation and self-replication via cloning. They continue the excision process of bodies deemed unworthy to appear among us and to share our world.[45] Perfection requires manipulation and elimination; there is a kind of purification imperative at work here as we aim to weed out the flawed and recognize only the perfect and fit. Wrapped up in a quest for control, immersed in the images and rhetoric of choice and self-possession, we will find it more and more difficult to ask the right sorts of questions as we will slowly but surely lose rich languages of opposition, like that embodied in Christian theological anthropology.

Notes

1. The United States is clearly my focus, although much if not all of what I say is applicable to the developed or, in John Paul II's terms, "super-developed cultures of consumption" of the West.

2. Abortion-on-demand at any stage of pregnancy and the death penalty would be the two prime candidates here. The paper's length is such that I will not be able to discuss these in full.

3. Dietrich Bonhoeffer, *Creation and Fall. A Theological Exposition of Genesis 1-3* (Minneapolis: Fortress Press, 1997). This is Volume 3 of *Dietrich Bonhoeffer Works*, now in progress.

4. This is not the time and the place to unpack ethical naturalism and moral realism. Suffice it to say that I am committed to the view that there is a 'there there,' that there are truths to be discerned about the world and that the world isn't just so much putty in our conceptually deft hands. The world exists independent of our minds but our minds possess the wonderful capacity to apprehend the world, up to a point given the fallibility of reason.

5. One example would be the work of philosopher, Judith Jarvis Thompson, known for her current support of physician assisted suicide, but who first made her reputation by providing justifications for abortion by analogizing from a woman hooked up during her sleep to a violinist for whom she was then required to provide life support, to a woman in relationship to the fetus she is carrying. Thompson claimed that the woman would be within her rights to unhook the violinist, even if it meant his or her death; similarly, a woman is not required to carry a fetus to term. I have never understood why a reasonable person would find this argument compelling. Fetuses do not get attached covertly but emerge as a result of action in which the woman is implicated. Furthermore, the fetus's dependence on the mother for sustenance for nine months is part of the order of nature—it simply is the way humans reproduce. There are many ways to sustain violinists in need of life support, and an adult violinist is scarcely analogous in any way to the life of a human being *in situ*.

6. Robin Lovin, *Niebuhr and Christian Realism*, p. 123.

7. Ibid., p. 126.

8. Ibid., p. 94.

9. Ibid., p. 130.

10. This, too, is more complex than simply acquiescence. For example, where the matter of abortion is concerned, there is enormous popular support for some forms of restriction and restraint on the practice. The elite culture (the media, those with incomes over $50,000 per year, lawyers, as the most reliable social science studies demonstrate) long ago fell into lock-step with an absolute abortion 'right,' including partial birth abortion, a practice the American Medical Association itself has declared not to be a legitimate medical procedure. So on the level of opinion all is not homogeneous. But this opinion rarely translates into action of any sort. Thus, the atrophy of civic habits of the past four

decades or so goes hand-in-hand with the triumph of projects that constitute flights from finitude.

11. Not ours alone, of course, but I will concentrate primarily on North American culture in depicting this obsession and grappling with its hold on the collective psyche.

12. Just to be clear at the outset, I do not intend to issue strictures against any and all attempts to intervene through modern forms of gene therapy in order to forestall, say, the development of devastating, inherited conditions or diseases. There is a huge difference between preventing an undeniable harm—say a type of inherited condition that dooms a child to a short and painful life—and striving to create a blemish-less perfect human specimen. How one differentiates the one from the other is part of the burden of argument. One example of justifiable intervention would be a method of gene therapy that spares children "the devastating effects of a rare but deadly inherited disease. In the condition, Crigler-Najjar syndrome, a substance called bilirubin, a waste product from the destruction of worn-out red blood cells, builds up in the body.... Bilirubin accumulates, causing jaundice, a yellowing of the skin and the whites of the eyes. More important, bilirubin is toxic to the nervous system, and the children live in constant danger of brain damage. The only way they can survive is to spend 10 to 12 hours a day under special lights that break down the bilirubin. But as they reach their teens, the light therapy becomes less effective. Unless they can get a liver transplant, they may suffer brain damage or die." Because previous attempts at gene therapy have all fallen far short of expectations, none of this may work. But it would spare a small number of children tremendous suffering and this sort of intervention is entirely defensive—it involves no eugenics ideology of any kind. See Denise Grady, "At Gene Therapy's Frontier, the Amish Build a Clinic," *The New York Times*, Science Times (Tuesday, June 29, 1999, pp. D1, 4), p. D1.

13. Cited in Roger Shattuck, *Forbidden Knowledge* (New York: Harcourt Brace, 1996), p. 1973.

14. As reprinted in an editorial in *Commonweal* (March 26, 1999, p. 5).

15. Ibid.

16. Doris T. Zallen, "We Need a Moratorium on 'Genetic Enhancement,' *The Chronicle of Higher Education* (March 27, 1998), p. A64.

17. James LeFanu, "Geneticists are not gods," *The Tablet* (12 December 1998, pp. 1645-1646), p. 1645.

18. Ibid.

19. A bit reminiscent of Julia, young female sexual revolutionary, in Orwell's *Brave New World*. She is, of course, defeated and comes to love Big Brother.

20. Hans S. Reinders, *The Future of the Disabled in Liberal Society: An Ethical Analysis* (Notre Dame: University of Notre Dame Press, 2000).

21. Please note that I do not want in any way to diminish the difficulties involved in parenting a child with disabilities. As the mother of an adult daughter with

mental retardation, I understand this very well. Instead, I am trying to capture the present temperament that dictates that such births are calamitous and ought never occur.

22. "Search and Destroy Missions," *U.S. Catholic* (January, 2000, p. 16).

23. Ibid.

24. Stephen S. Hall, "The Recycled Generation," *The New York Times Magazine* (January 30, 2000, pp. 30-35, 46, 74-79.)

25. Ibid., p.32.

26. But who defines excess? This is a squishy soft criterion that now comes into play at present for such 'abnormalities' as cleft palate.

27. Quoted from the *Journal of Engineering and Science* in Shattuck, *Forbidden Knowledge*, pp. 193-194. The literature of reportage, enthusiasm, concern, *et. al.*, is nearly out of control. A few magazine and newspaper pieces worth reading include: Jim Yardley, "Investigators Say Embryologist Knew He Erred in Egg Mix-Up," *The New York Times* (Saturday, April 17, 1999), p. A13; Martin Lupton, "Test-tube questions," *The Tablet* (20 February 1999), pp. 259-260; David L. Marcus, "Mothers with another's eggs," *U .S. News and World Report* (April 13, 1999), pp. 42-44; Nicholas Wade, "Panel Told of Vast Benefits of Embryo Cells," *The New York Times* (Thursday, December 3, 1998, p. A24); Anne Taylor Fleming, "Why I Can't Use Someone Else's Eggs," *Newsweek* (April 12, 1999), p. 12; Nicholas Wade, "Gene Study Bolsters Hope for Treating Diseases of Aging," *The New York Times* (Friday, March 5, 1999, p. A12); Lisa Belkiun, "Splice Einstein and Sammy Glick. Add a Little Magellan," *The New York Times Magazine* (August 23, 1998, pp. 26-31, 56-61). A chilling piece that shows the many ways in which gene-enthusiasm and commodification fuse; "Stephanie Armour, "Could your genes hold you back?" *USA Today* (Wednesday, May 5, 1999, pp. B1-2). An example of how the bizarre becomes commonplace is Gina Kolata, "Scientists Place Jellyfish Genes into Monkeys," *The New York Times* (Thursday, December 23, 1999, pp. 1-20.) We have normalized the preposterous and do not even ask: why on earth would anyone do that—put jellyfish genes into monkeys?

28. The article begins on p. 1 and continues on page A17 of the *Times* for that day.

29. This foreboding also comes through in Bryan Appleyard, *Brave New Worlds. Staying Human in the Genetic Future* (New York: Viking, 1998.)

30. I cannot here deal with the commercialization of genetics but the huge profits to be made drive much of the scientific and technological work, alas. See, for example, Lisa Belkin, "Splice Einstein and Sammy Glick. Add a Little Magellan," *New York Times Magazine* (August 23, 1998, pp. 26-31.)

31. Think, by the way, of what this would have done to Martin Luther King's protest: simply stopped it dead in the tracks. For the law of the Jim Crow South was the law of segregation. And no ethical argument can challenge the law. End of story. A comeback would be that you need to make a legal argument to change the law. But King's call for legal change was an ethical call. The reduc-

tive argument that law and ethics must never touch is a crude form of legal positivism, or command-obedience legal theory. What is right doesn't enter into the picture at all.

32. Pontifical Academy for Life, "Reflections on Cloning," *Origins* (May 21, 1998, Vol. 28, No. 1, pp.14-16), p. 15. The popular press has been filled with cloning articles. A few include, Sheryl WuDunn, "South Korean Scientists Say They Cloned a Human Cell," *The New York Times* (Thursday, December 17, 1998, p. A12); Nicholas Wade, "Researchers Join in Effort On Cloning Repair Tissue," *The New York Times* (Wednesday, May 5, 1999, p. A19), p. A19; Tim Friend, "Merger could clone bio-companies' creativity," *USA Today* (Wednesday, May 5, 1999, p. 13A). See also Lori B. Andrews, *The Clone Age. Adventures in the New World of Reproductive Technology* (New York: Henry Holt, 1999).

33. But we have a solution to that one, too, don't we? We can be certain that the creatures nobody wants, whose lives are not "worth living," can be easily dispatched to spare their suffering. Physician-assisted suicide, the track down which we are moving, is, of course, part and parcel of the general tendencies I here discuss and criticize. Although I do not focus specifically on this matter, I recommend the following two essays for the general reader: Paul R. McHugh, "The Kevorkian Epidemic," *The American Scholar* (Winter, 1997, pp. 15-27); Leon R. Kass and Nelson Lund, "Courting Death: Assisted Suicide, Doctors, and the Law," *Commentary* (December, 1996, pp. 17-29); and, as well, the late Cardinal Bernardin's "Letter to the Supreme Court," which was appended to a friend-of-the-court brief filed by the Catholic Health Association in a Supreme Court case testing the appeals of two lower court decisions that struck down laws prohibiting assisted suicide in Washington and New York States; and a brief by the U.S. Catholic Conference, "Assisted Suicide Issue Moves to Supreme Court," *Origins* (December 12, 1996, Vol. 26, No. 26 , pp. 421-430.)

34. Leon R. Kass, "The Wisdom of Repugnance," *The New Republic* (June 2, 1997, pp. 17-26), p. 20.

35. There is a big discussion here yearning to breathe free, of course, namely, the connection between beauty and truth. But it is one I cannot even begin to enter on at this point. The truth is often described as splendid and beautiful— Augustine's language—and God as beautiful in and through God's simplicity. The aesthetic dimension in theology and, most certainly in ethics, is underexplored.

36. Kass, "The Wisdom of Repugnance," p. 20.

37. *Ibid.*, p. 21.

38. *Ibid.*, pp. 22-24.

39. See Roger Shattuck's wonderful discussion of Faust and Frankenstein in his *Forbidden Knowledge* (New York: Harcourt Brace, Harvest Book), 1996.

40. *Original Unity*, p. 23.

41. Karol Wojtyla, *Sign of Contradiction* (New York: Seabury, 1979), p. 24.

42. *Ibid.*, p. 124.

43. This discussion in Bonhoeffer's *Ethics* appears on pp.142-185 and all quoted matter is drawn from those pages inclusively.

44. This is an area that deserves longer treatment than I can here give it. Fortunately, and at long last, there are texts in English on Nazi euthanasia as part of its general bio-politics. Of especial note is Michael Burleigh, *Death and Deliverance* (Cambridge: Cambridge University Press, 1994). This is a tremendously disquieting book for a contemporary American reader. So much of the language of our own genetic engineering and "assisted suicide" proponents seems echoes of National Socialist propaganda. The Nazis covered the waterfront, so to speak, justifying their programs of systematic selective elimination of the "unfit," of life unworthy of life (congenitally 'diseased', handicapped, etc.) on a number of interrelated grounds, including cost-benefit criteria, perfecting the race, and compassion. The Nazis also controlled the media on this issue (it goes without saying), producing short propaganda films and full-length features, lavishly produced and starring German matinee idols, to promote their euthanasia efforts.

45. In a longer paper, the death penalty would come under critical scrutiny here as an act of such radical excision.

CHAPTER 3

The Magisterium on the Cutting Edge: Evangelization and Culture

John M. Haas

The man across the table from me was articulate, passionate, zealous, brilliant, principled, and committed to doing good. I sat spellbound as he delivered for my personal benefit one of the most fascinating and lucid microbiology lectures I had ever heard. He was also engaged in research that I found absolutely morally reprehensible.

His company, Advanced Cell Technology, was taking the DNA from human somatic cells, placing it in e-nucleated cows' eggs and beginning the cloning process for a human being. The organism would be allowed to grow to a mass of about 100 cells before it would be dissected to obtain human embryonic stem cells for research. These were cloned human beings with cow mitochondrial genetic material mingled in.

The company had no interest in producing cross-species creatures. Its activities were driven by concerns of simple research, efficiency, and cost control. For the cloning process, cows eggs were easier and cheaper to obtain than human ova. Also, the cow's eggs were bigger than human ova and easier to work with. These were utilitarian concerns, pure and simple.

But while we spoke in his *boardroom*, in his *laboratories* human embryos were lying in Petri dishes, subjected to experimentation, dissected and killed, and frozen for future use. Human embryos. Embryonic human beings. It does not matter how it is put, they were beings that were human.

Poet, apostle, philosopher, theologian, bard and playwright within our cultural tradition once spoke of the transcendent worth and inviolability of our kind, of the human being. Legislators, jurists, warriors, and police once protected the innocent of our species from the first moment of conception. The medical profession from the time of the pagan Hippocrates swore never to kill the unborn child. In more recent times, the World Medical Association adopted the *Declaration of Geneva*, which includes an oath for physicians to take upon beginning their medical career in which they vow, "I will maintain the utmost respect for human life, from the time of conception."

It was *human* life that engendered such awe, the creature before whom we stood in reverence, for in this creature we saw even more than ourselves. We could see the very image of God Himself. We were not simply one species among others. As the psalmist and later the apostle would declare, "What is man, O Lord, that you are mindful of him, the son of man that you care for him? You have made him a little lower than the angels; you have crowned him with glory and honor, subjecting all things under his feet."[1]

The bard and playwright Shakespeare declared with equal eloquence, "What a piece of work is man, how noble in reason, how infinite in faculties…in action how like an angel, in apprehension how like a god: the beauty of the world, the paragon of animals…."[2]

But it was man's Godlike qualities that set him apart from the rest of creation. His dignity was a participatory dignity, for One alone is truly good, the One in whose image we had been created and by whom we had been redeemed. That living reality which engendered such reverence now lies in untold numbers of Petri dishes. Those formerly awe-inspiring beings are now experimented upon, dissected, and cloned. They are frozen in suspended animation, in countless containers of liquid nitrogen. Man has been increasingly stripped of his Godlike qualities even as he presumes to act more and more like God. One of the developers of in vitro fertilization has declared that it is a sin to bring a deformed child into the world. But the God whom we worship is described thus:

> "There were many who were astonished at him—so marred was his appearance…"[3]
> "He had no form or majesty that we should look at him, nothing in his appearance that we should desire him…a man of suffering and acquainted with infirmity…."[4]

That is the God of whom we had stood in awe and whom we would see and venerate in the weakest, the sickest, and the most vulnerable.

Now, in our contemporary culture of death, these are the very ones who are viewed as expendable, as the source of cells, tissue, and organs for the benefit of others. It is the overarching philosophy of abject materialism that has robbed man of his dignity. The supposed material origins of human life are not even questioned in our day. The Princeton molecular biologist Lee Silver states baldly what he believes to be the truth, "…most biologists believe that life had to coalesce spontaneously from inanimate matter on earth."[5] Yet, the truly unreasonable position is that this creature "noble in reason…infinite in faculties" could have spontaneously arisen from inanimate matter. Yet, the materialism that strips the human person of his transcendent meaning dominates our cultural consciousness.

In truth, we cannot properly speak of man without speaking of the One who has created him. In fact, without his creator man is, quite fundamentally, unintelligible.

In his book, *Existentialism*, the atheist Jean Paul Sartre says there is no human nature because there is no God to creatively conceive it. The Catholic German philosopher Josef Pieper maintained that Sartre's logic was unassailable. If Sartre's premise were accepted, i.e., that there is no God, then his conclusion would naturally follow that there is no human nature. Pieper pointed out that anything has a nature by virtue of its having been created. A pair of eyeglasses are eyeglasses precisely because that is what they were created to be. The creator of anything bestows the nature upon what has been created. If there is no Creator God, then there is no human nature as such. Human beings would simply be so much raw material, so much stuff, to be manipulated and used, redirected and reconstituted at the whim of those who had power over them.

In our civilization, human dignity, and the safeguards put in place to acknowledge and protect that dignity, was derived primarily from the recognition of a Creator. Innocent human life was sacred because the One in whose image it was created was known and acknowledged as sacred.

However, today we live in a society which is so de-sacralized, so secularized, that nothing is sacred any longer, not even innocent human life. In fact, not only is human life no longer regarded as sacred, it is no longer even understood for what it is. Having lost sight of God, we no longer understand even who or what man is. Medical science now treats man in a manner similar to veterinary medicine dealing with lower animals. Contraceptive and reproductive techniques, some of which have been around for centuries, have never been applied to human beings until our own day. Camel drivers on caravans wanted to prevent the female camels from becoming pregnant during the trek across the desert. So, they would simply thrust a stone up into the uterus. Centuries later in America, we thrust IUD's into a woman's uterus, a technique long used on camels. Cats are spayed and dogs neutered, now we do it to human beings. Artificial insemination has long been standard in the breeding of cattle. We now do it to women. Horses are put out of their misery after breaking a leg. We now do it to human beings. Human life in its coming into being is no longer considered human life and is subjected to experimentation and the ignominy of cryopreservation. We no longer treat human beings with the awe and reverence due to those endowed with the divine image. The words of the Second Vatican Council have proven to be prophetic in our own day, "When God is forgotten . . .the creature itself grows unintelligible."[6]

When Karol Woytila wrote his first encyclical as Pope John Paul II, he dedicated it to the human person and warned of the implications of this practical atheism to be found in the West of which I have been speaking:

Man's situation in the modern world seems indeed to be far removed from the objective demands of the moral order, from the requirements of justice, and even more of social love. We are dealing here only with that which found expression in the Creator's first message to man at the moment in which He was giving him the earth, to 'subdue' it. This first message was confirmed by Christ the Lord in the mystery of the Redemption...The essential meaning of this 'kingship' and 'dominion' of man over the visible world, which the Creator Himself gave man for his task, consists in the priority of ethics over technology, in the primacy of the person over things, and in the superiority of spirit over matter.[7]

As the English cultural historian Christopher Dawson put it in his *Progress and Religion,* "It is the religious impulse which supplies the cohesive force which unifies a society and a culture.... A society which has lost its religion becomes sooner or later a society which has lost its soul." And when the soul of a society has been lost, it is man himself who ultimately suffers. As Pope John Paul II has said: "We have before us here a great drama that can leave nobody indifferent. The person who, on the one hand, is trying to draw the maximum profit and, on the other hand, is paying the price in damage and injury, *is always man.*"[8]

What has this meant for man as the biotech century dawns? A myriad of new ways have developed for engendering human life and many result in man paying the price in damage and injury, even as he tries to draw the maximum profit. Surrogate mothers are often indigent women who are willing to subject themselves to artificial insemination, to the dangers of pregnancy, and to the relinquishing of their rights and obligations toward their own child for the fee, which is earned through the procedure. To ensure a greater chance of a successful pregnancy through in vitro fertilization, several embryos are engendered. Only the healthy survive the Petri dish. Once a number of embryos have been implanted in the woman's womb, only one of them will usually survive so-called "fetal reduction." What appear to be good and noble undertakings result in the wastage of human life and in a violation of the integrity of marriage.

When I met with the head of Advance Cell Technology who was cloning humans with cow eggs and human DNA, he was amazed to learn that the Catholic Church had actually condemned cloning humans in 1987. The Congregation for the Doctrine of the Faith had issued an "instruction" which morally assessed various means of overcoming infertility. One reason for his amazement was the fact that the Holy See had condemned cloning at a time when the scientific community thought that the cloning of mammals was impossible. *Donum Vitae* was issued in 1987, ten years before the first cloning of a mammal, the sheep Dolly. At the same time, the Holy See condemned the engendering of human life through parthenogenesis, a technique which has been developed, albeit not yet successfully, in only the last few months.

How is it that the magisterium of the Catholic Church was able to anticipate and morally assess a means of engendering life before it had even been developed? How is it equipped to reflect morally on human developments even before they occur?

The magisterium of the Church can accomplish this because the Church is, as Pope Paul VI said, "the expert in humanity." The Church knows human nature, in its created state, in its fallen condition, and in its redeemed state. The Church knows whence man has come from and whither he is going. She knows this without any doubt or confusion. The Church knows the purposes for which man was created, and so she can unerringly judge whether certain actions will thwart those purposes or help man to achieve them.

It is fundamentally impossible to address the ethical issues of reproductive technologies, cloning, or stem cell research without seeing that the debates surrounding these issues take place in a cultural context, a context that fundamentally shapes the debate itself and gives meaning to the words being used. The truth is that in any society there is always a dominant view of the world, which frames the debates and which is so pervasive that it is not even questioned.

There are certain cultural presuppositions in our own society that are the starting points for conversation, for public policy, and for our common life. These presuppositions function as kinds of cultural coordinates that help navigate society from one point to the next. They are not questioned any more than sailors would question the position of the stars by which they navigate from port to port. There are indeed a number of such cultural coordinates, and the ones most prominent in our society go by the names of moral relativism, utilitarianism, and human autonomy. I suppose the one word that has come to embody them all in popular culture is "Choice." I will choose whether I live or die—and if you are sufficiently weak and vulnerable and dependent, I will choose whether YOU live or die.

Our Holy Father gave us a remarkably insightful encyclical a few years ago entitled *Evangelium Vitae* or *The Gospel of Life*. Some people hailed this encyclical as a tremendous advance in the development of moral teaching, since the encyclical moved very close to making infallible pronouncements on the direct killing of the innocent, on abortion and euthanasia.

I would submit that the encyclical is indeed a clear, forceful, and unequivocal teaching on the immorality of abortion and euthanasia. But, it cannot be seen as an advance since that teaching has always been in place, both in the hearts of men, as St. Paul reminds us in Romans, as well as in the written word of God, "Thou shalt not murder." The intention of the Encyclical *The Gospel of Life* was to provide a penetrating reflection upon and analysis of the underlying cultural presuppositions that have given rise to what the Holy Father has called, "The Culture of Death." The encyclical is fundamentally a critique of culture, our culture, an advanced technological and secularized culture. The Pope poses more a cultural question than a moral one when he asks in the encyclical, "How is it possible that what was abhorred as a crime in very recent history has now come to be claimed as a human right? How is it possible?"

What has happened culturally is that a liberal Protestant, Enlightenment, and secularist worldview has become dominant in our society and has suppressed any mode of discourse that acknowledges the spiritual, the transcendent, the supernatural, and the divine. As a consequence, it is impossible to understand what is the true nature of the human person, who even in his natural state is the image of the ineffable God who has created him. Remember that it is an insight of natural reason, not just divine revelation, that there is a God who has created the world—which is by virtue of that creation intelligible and predictable. It also means that there is an objective moral order to which man must conform if he would find true happiness.

As Catholics we are not surprised that individuals are trying to accomplish great good through many of these new procedures in the so-called "reproductive technologies." Although even to use the term reproductive instead of procreative and to apply the notion of technologies to the engendering of new human life, vividly illustrate the dehumanization of the human person which has occurred in our secularized, Godless culture.

But as Catholics we ought not to be surprised that individuals are trying to accomplish good through these procedures to overcome infertility or other problems inherent in generating new life. This does not surprise us because the Catholic Church actually espouses a very positive philosophical anthropology, or understanding of the human person. The doctrine of "the total depravity of man" is not of our religious tradition. We believe that what fundamentally drives human behavior is a search for happiness and a desire to do good.

People never cease to be amazed when they actually encounter the Catholic understanding of sin. When I met with the other scientists at Advanced Cell Technology, I pointed out that the *Catechism of the Catholic Church* does not define sin fundamentally as an act against God's will or His commandments or His laws. The *Catechism of the Catholic Church* teaches that "sin is an offense against reason, truth and right conscience; it is failure in genuine love for God and neighbor caused by a perverse attachment to certain goods."[9] The scientist who had been cloning himself by using cells from the inside of his cheek exclaimed, "Wow, sin as an act against reason!" He began writing down the quote and asked, "Who said that again?" To his incredulity I pointed out again that it was the teaching of the Catholic Church.

But it should be noted that the understanding of sin within the Catholic tradition sees the act as not only "an act against reason" but also as "a perverse attachment to certain goods." The anthropology of our religious tradition is such that we see even in human sin a natural human attachment to "certain goods." Catholics are not surprised when they are told by those whom they are trying to dissuade from immoral actions that these individuals are only trying to do good. This is what we understand to be the motivation for human behavior.

The biotech researcher wants to obtain embryonic stem cells, which are pluripotent, to see if he is able to tease them into becoming neurological cells to help cure Alzheimers or Parkinsons Disease. He has no particular ghoulish pleasure in destroying human embryos. The physician sets about to abort the encephalic child because he wants to help the parents avoid an emotionally wrenching and difficult birth and early death, not because he hates children. The fertility technician engenders *eight* embryos in Petri dishes, instead of just one, in order to increases the chances that a couple will be able to overcome their heartbreaking infertility. The surrogate mother who already has two children of her own is willing to endure the difficulties of another pregnancy in order to help an infertile couple have their own child—or to make more money for her own family. Reproductive scientists feel badly for the lesbian couple unable to have a child of their own genetic make-up, so they devise a technique to make this possible. Pre-implantation genetic diagnosis is used in order to avoid implanting a child that will be a hemophiliac.

The Catholic is not surprised by the great good all these individuals want to bring about. In fact, he expects that they will be so motivated. The task of the Church, her magisterium, and of each individual Catholic is to bring these people to see that even as they want to do good things, the means they are choosing may themselves not be good. In fact, the means may be wretchedly evil because they assault fundamental human goods. The heart of the immoral behavior is not that these people are seeking to do evil, and it certainly is not that these individuals have an attachment to certain goods, but rather that the attachment to the goods they seek is disordered in some way.

The fundamental moral principle that applies to bioethics is the same one that applies to economics, theories of a just war, medicine, and social communications. "Primum non nocere." First of all, "Do no harm." All of the actions proposed earlier, the abortion, the in vitro fertilization, are meant to enhance human happiness, human flourishing. There is the desire to have children when it is not possible or to avoid children when having them would appear to hurt someone. There is the burning wish to save lives or to overcome crippling pathologies. There is, in a word, a desire to promote human flourishing. The one thing that must be avoided in that pursuit is anything that would diminish human flourishing, that would denigrate human goods, which would violate human dignity because it would vitiate the very good being sought.

The resolution of these dreadful social and moral evils will be accomplished only through the re-evangelization of culture, so that we can once again come to know the true nature of the human person, of marital love, and of establishing and raising families. Many of the activities taking place within the so-called biotechnology industry and many of the attitudes which are fostered toward the human person within that industry, put the lie to the good that is sought.

Great human good can come from contemporary advances in microbiology and biochemistry, but these advances will turn to bitter ash if they are achieved at the expense of the human person. This human embryo lying in a Petri dish was created a little lower than the angels and is destined to be crowned in glory and honor. To destroy it, to experiment upon it, and to use if for the benefit of others is to violate its dignity and frankly the dignity of those who would so use it. The Church teaches us in *Donum Vitae*:

> the fruit of human generation, from the first moment of its existence, that is to say, from the moment the zygote has formed, demands the unconditional respect that is morally due to the human being in his bodily and spiritual totality. The human being is to be respected and treated as a person from the moment of conception; and therefore from that same moment his rights as a person must be recognized, among which in the first place is the inviolable right of every innocent human being to life.[10]

Pope John Paul II writes, "This century has so far been a century of great calamities for man, of great devastations, not only material ones but also moral ones, indeed, perhaps above all, moral ones."[11] This new Century may be one of new human hope if Catholics enthusiastically undertake the re-evangelization of culture under the teaching and governing authority of the magisterium.

Notes

1. Hebrews 2:6-8
2. William Shakespeare, *Hamlet*, 2.2.
3. Is. 52:14
4. Is. 52:2-3
5. Lee M. Silver, *Remaking Eden: Cloning and Beyond in a Brave New World* (New York: Avon Books, 1997), 28.
6. Pastoral Constitution on the Church in the Modern World, *Gaudium et Spes*, 36.
7. John Paul II, *Redemptor Hominis*, 16.
8. Ibid.
9. Libreria Editrice Vaticana, *Catechism of the Catholic Church* (Washington, DC: United States Catholic Conference, 1997), 1849.
10. Congregation for the Doctrine of Faith, *Donum Vitae Part I: Respect for Human Embryos* (1987), 1.
11. John Paul II, *Redemptor Hominis*, 17.

CHAPTER 4

Human Dignity and Reproductive Technology: Pastoral Implications

Steven Bozza

Infertility is a growing phenomenon. At the beginning of the new millennium, roughly 20% of couples of childbearing age will experience difficulty conceiving. There are a number of reasons for this situation. Some cases arise from the choices couples make to marry later in life and delay childbirth. Other cases are the direct result of sexually transmitted diseases. Sometimes environmental hazards wreak havoc on the reproductive system, and still other cases may stem from physiological problems (e.g., endometriosis). Approximately 14% of infertility cases are simply unexplained. Regardless of the causes of infertility, the percentages of couples with this problem are higher today than in the past.

Medical science has responded to this decrease in fertility rates by developing a vast array of reproductive technologies. Because of the highly technical nature of these developments, many couples do not understand the medical treatments offered to them and are often at the mercy of health care professionals who more than likely place scientific advancement above theological and philosophical arguments to the contrary. To complicate matters further, most couples are either uninformed or misinformed regarding the Church's teaching on the truth and meaning of human sexuality.

The Catholic Church has been at the forefront of moral deliberations regarding assisted fertility treatment. For the Church, it is the dignity of the human person, marriage, and the marital act, which is the basis of Her moral determinations. She looks to what is natural, the natural law, in order to determine which techniques are morally sound and which are not.

Along with the objective moral truths concerning infertility treatments, there are a myriad of subjective realities, which might make a morally acceptable procedure unacceptable to an individual couple. And so, the pastoral care of couples experiencing infertility must be holistic. It must not only concern itself with the morality of the biological procedures, but also with the psychological, social, and spiritual issues which such couples face.

A Devastating Reality

"As an incarnate spirit, that is a soul which expresses itself in a body and a body informed by an immortal spirit, man is called to love in his unified totality."[1] Sexuality is a part of human personhood, an inseparable component of the intellect. Human persons, infused with a male or female soul, think and act through the lens of their sexuality. Thus, "femininity and masculinity are complementary gifts through which human sexuality is an integrating part of the concrete capacity to love which God has inscribed in man and woman."[2] This gives the body a nuptial meaning because of its capacity to love as self-giving.[3]

> In its most profound reality, love is essentially a gift; and conjugal love, while leading the spouses to the reciprocal "knowledge"…does not end with the couple, because it makes them capable of the greatest possible gift, the gift by which they become cooperators with God for giving life to a new human person. Thus, the couple, while giving themselves to one another, give not just themselves but also the reality of children, who are living reflection of their love, a permanent sign of conjugal unity and a living and inseparable synthesis of their being father and a mother.[4]

Thus, infertility strikes at the heart of a marital identity. It shakes the inner core of the human person. Masculinity and fatherhood and femininity and motherhood are not merely descriptive words. They are often intertwined realities, which mean the same thing to many people.

Human sexuality, as a gift given by God, allows the human person to share in God's life. It is oriented to "relationship" and is a gift to be given and to be received. Infertility, therefore, strikes not only at a person's self image, but also at the couple's relationship.

How then can we best help couples come to terms with infertility? First, we must first walk with them through each of the stages of denial, anger, frustration, pain, jealousy, and confusion. The pain, guilt, and poor self-image that accompany infertility are similar to the suffering caused by the death of a loved one. The loved one in this case is the child yet to be conceived. The couple loves the child even though he or she does not exist. To return to wholeness, the couple must grieve properly for the loss of the one they love.

Grieving is a process. Each stage is important and necessary. The hopelessness, questioning, anger, and feelings of abandonment are not signs of a weak faith. They are a part of the process that God allows in order to work through the difficult and painful experiences of life.

The Stages of Grief

Shock and Disbelief. The haunting question that a couple will often ask is, "why has this happened to us?" Throughout their lives, men and women prepare for parenthood. In experiencing their father's expression of fatherhood, boys learn how or how not to be a father. The same holds true for girls, who learn how or how not to be a mother by experiencing their mother's expression of motherhood. As individuals and as a couple, hopeful parents dream of their children's names, the special events, and their aspirations for them. When infertility disrupts these hopes, their dreams are shattered.

Anger and Resentment. Couples coping with infertility often experience anger, resentment, and jealousy toward others with children, toward their spouses, and even toward God. Often they will avoid social gatherings such as baby showers or Christenings in an attempt to avoid the pain of infertility. They may sometimes blame their spouses, which more often than not reflects the pain of an increasingly deteriorating self-image. Even God is not immune to the couple's anger and resentment. They question God's love for them and His concern for their needs.

Despair and Depression. Following the feelings of disbelief and anger, many couples begin to give up hope when all seems to point to the inevitable, that the couple will simply not conceive. An overwhelming sense of loneliness and isolation ensues. Suddenly, their voices echo within the walls of their homes. They feel isolated from their parishes whose activities quite often revolve around family activities, the school, and youth ministries. Many times, couples experiencing infertility bury themselves in either their work or sensual pursuits to take their minds off parenthood.

Panic. During this stage, couples often scurry to find one last-ditch approach to conception. It may become an obsession, which has the potential to overshadow every part of their lives. When this happens, they no longer live in freedom. Rather, they enter into a form of slavery whereby all their activity is focused on this one goal.

Guilt. In the process of answering the question "why is this happening to us?" undoubtedly, the husband or wife, or maybe even both, will examine their past in an attempt to identify sins that, to them, warrant God's punishment. Particularly, past sexual sins are often the blame for present infertility. With these thoughts, a tremendous amount of guilt and remorse descends upon them. They feel ashamed because they aren't able to give either their spouse a child or their parents grandchildren.

Acceptance. Only after the experiences of shock, anger, despair, panic, and guilt can the couple come to acknowledge that they can live without children of their own. This does not mean they will be free from the pain that accompanies infertility. They may never be freed from it. Yet, the day will come when they are able to accept their situation.

Hope. At this stage, couples begin to dream again and re-vision their lives together. The pain of their suffering has moved them closer together because in a most profound way, they have entered more deeply into the mystery of each other. Their suffering has meaning because now their vision of a future together is forged from a common refiner's fire.

Vocation

After a couple reaches the stage of hope and begins to re-vision their future, the pastoral care worker must build within them a sense of vocation as individuals and as a couple. Having children is sometimes considered the only vocation a marriage can have. Forgotten are the other gifts married couples give to each other and to those around them.

The primary vocation of all human persons is to love as God loves. His is a self-emptying love, which brings forth abundant life. Marriage is a vocation to self-giving love whereby a man and a woman continue the flow of love to life. They are no longer spectators in God's creative process, instead they are participators. This is the highest vocation of married couples: to give their love names and to give to God these new lives. However, this vocation to generate new lives for God has not been given to some. Does this mean their marriage is deficient? That it has no meaning? Certainly not.

Having children is not the only vocation within a marriage. All married couples give life to each other. They do this by affirming each other's goodness and by encouraging each other to be all that God wants them to be.

Along with being life-giving to each other, as a couple they are called to be life-giving to those around them. They become spiritually fruitful to others enriching them with the gifts unique to their marriage. The duty of being life-giving to others is a part of their marital vocation. Discovering what this vocation is will provide meaning and purpose to their marriage.

Children are Gifts, Not Rights

The next step in the pastoral care of the couple is to help them understand that having a child is not a right, it is a privilege. For a woman, the supreme gift she can give to her husband is to bear his child. For a man, the supreme gift he can give to his wife is a child to love and nurture. When it is not possible to give this gift, the couple may feel deprived of the greatest act of love known to them.

This sense of deprivation may change their understanding of the meaning of a child. Being deprived of the gift of a child seems unfair to them. This feeling of unfairness may cause the couple to think that the child is actually a right. Yet, the greatest dignity of the child rests in the fact that he or she is an independent human being. The couple runs the risk of devaluing the dignity of the child if they conclude that he or she is a marital right. "Marriage does not confer upon the spouses the right to have a child, but only the right to perform those natural acts which are per se ordered to procreation."[5] Sadly, an extreme desire for children may progress to the point that the child becomes a commodity.[6]

The Good of the Couple

Lastly, we must review with the couple all the techniques that are available. We must help them to understand why some techniques are morally sound, why some are not, and why the circumstances of their lives may make a morally acceptable technique unacceptable to an individual couple. All this must be done in light of their inherent dignity as human persons.

Couples seeking a child will go to great lengths to conceive one. They often undergo humiliating forms of testing and treatment, which tear away at their dignity. They accept large financial burdens, which they carry for years. They endure the stress that enters their marriage and their marriage bed. They even risk the health hazards associated with fertility drugs and therapies. They do all of this with the idea that it will be worth it when they are finally able to carry their own child. But is it worth it? In most cases, it is not. Couples become blinded to these realities in their quest for a child until they cannot ignore them any longer. They lose sight of the true purpose of marriage and children, which threatens the dignity of both the couple and the greatly desired child.

Addressing the Issues

The examination of Scripture is essential in helping couples to understand the true nature and purpose of marriage and children.

> God created man in His image; in the divine image He created him; male and female He created them. God blessed them saying "Be fertile and multiply; fill the earth and subdue it. Have dominion over the fish of the sea, the birds of the air, and all the living things that move on the earth.[7]

Human persons are not spectators in God's creative plan, instead they are active participators. To be made in His image and likeness is to be a free rational being who gives love and receives love reciprocally.

The creation of man and woman, that is, the creation of humanity was one act. The second chapter of Genesis gives an account of creation that begins with the formation of man from the "clay of the earth"[8] and proceeds to state that "it is not good for the man to be alone."[9] At this point in the second creation story, the essence of both man and woman existed in *H'adam*—the man.[10]

It was only when Adam's solitude reached a crescendo that a suitable helpmate was presented to Him as a gift.[11] The man had to discover for himself that in order to be true to his identity as the enfleshed image of God, he needed to be able to express love through his body and become one flesh with another person. Thus, the woman was not an afterthought. Only after the division of the sexes was *H'adam* self-defined as *ish*—the male. The woman was defined in *relationship* to him *ishah*[12] "for out of her man this one was taken."[13]

Only after this dynamic is understood can the deeply intimate vocation to be co-creators with God be put in its proper perspective. God did it once and inscribed it within the human heart to participate and continue in His creative process until the earth is full with His children.

He also gave to man all of creation in its raw beauty and majesty. Through the properties of the human soul, the gifts of creativity, wisdom, and art, men and women, by the work of their hands, are called to refine and perfect creation and leave within it a human face.

In a fallen world, the perfection of creation is most often combined with the destruction of it, and so subduing the earth and having dominion over creation takes on an added meaning. Humanity is called to overcome natural difficulties and find ways of curing illness and disease. In the consideration of reproductive technology, this duty is best understood in a series of building blocks.

Building Block 1: By virtue of our call to subdue the earth and to have dominion over creation, infertility treatment per se is morally acceptable.

The Objective Moral Order

The Lord God then took the man and settled him in the Garden of Eden, to cultivate and care for it. The Lord God gave man this order: "You are free to eat from any of the trees of the garden except the Tree of Knowledge of Good and Bad. From that tree you shall not eat; the moment you eat from it you are surely doomed to die."[14]

Human freedom is far reaching. "You are free to eat from any of the trees of the garden." But it is not without limits "except from the Tree of the Knowledge of Good and Evil."[15] The consequences of going beyond the parameters set by God are stark—death and destruction. This sets up the whole objective moral order.

In regard to human reproduction, marriage and married love are by nature ordered to the procreation and education of children.[16] Thus, the freedom to find ways to overcome infertility must be rooted in marriage and have as its source the language of love, the marital act. Any act or procedure outside marriage and the marital act will lead to the destruction of human dignity and human life.

Building Block 2:The first step in discernment is to eliminate all objectively evil therapy and procedures. They are:

1. A.I.D.—Artificial insemination using donor gametes.
2. I.V.F.—Invitro fertilization

3. Z.I.F.T.—Zygote intrafallopian transfer
4. I.C.S.I.—Introcytoplasmic sperm injection, a form of I.V.F.
5. Cloning
6. Surrogacy
7. Embryo cryopreservation
8. Multifetal pregnancy reduction—a procedure in which the number of gestational sacs is reduced. This procedure is used to decrease the number of fetuses a woman carries and thereby improve the chances that the remaining fetuses will survive and develop into healthy infants.

Subjective Realities

In discerning the type and extent of infertility treatment, the following subjective factors must be considered:

1. The Dignity of the Man and the Woman

The nature and intensity of infertility testing and treatment affects the most private and personal parts of the body and psyche. This may not bother every couple, however, many feel violated in either some or all of the procedures.

The testing and therapy may cause physical or emotional trauma, which can affect the couple's health and their relationships. If this happens, their dignity and bodily integrity are compromised.

Building Block 3: If their dignity as persons is eroding because of their decision to pursue morally acceptable infertility treatment options, then these options may not be morally acceptable to the couple.

2. The Dignity of Their Marriage

The stress and regimen of infertility therapy can become intense. It can shake the stability of even the strongest of marriages. They may place high expectations on their spouses to do more than he or she is willing to do to achieve their dream of a child. Their love and desire for each other can very easily become overshadowed by their love and desire for this yet to be conceived child. This may lead to a disintegration of their relationship.

Building Block 4: If their marriage relationship is suffering because of their decision to pursue morally acceptable infertility treatment options, then these options may not be morally acceptable to the couple.

3. The Dignity of Their Marital Act

Throughout the process of trying to conceive a child, sexual intercourse may be less an act of love and self-giving and more a clinical act. When the time of sexual expression becomes "baby making" and not "lovemaking," it can cause harm to them as a man or as a woman. When they experience a shift of attitude from lover and beloved to function and performance, the unifying significance of the marital act is lost and disunity may follow.

Building Block 5: If their marital act is more often than not a clinical act because of their decision to pursue morally acceptable infertility treatment options, then these options may not be morally acceptable for the couple.

4. The Stability of Their Finances

The cost of infertility testing and treatments is quite high. Some of them are covered by insurance. Many of them are not. Since there is a success rate of 25%–35% for most Assisted Fertility Technology, multiple attempts to affect conception must take place. Is the couple getting into excessive debt to conceive a child? Is the money they are spending on this project more urgently needed elsewhere?

Building Block 6: If the stability of their finances is threatened and if they run the risk of not being a good steward of their resources because of their decision to pursue morally acceptable infertility treatment options, then these options may not be morally acceptable for the couple.

Making Decisions

Making medical decisions is never an easy task. In any such decision, the focus should be on healing the whole person. A truly healthy person is one whose body is working properly, whose mind is functioning optimally, whose spirit is oriented to God, and whose social relationships are in order. Because of the nature of infertility testing and treatments, this holistic approach to decision making becomes all the more important.

Thus, in the decision making process, **the first step** is to rule out the options that violate the objective moral order. These are the procedures that the couple can never undergo.

The second step is to evaluate the subjective realities in the couple's life, which can make a morally acceptable procedure unacceptable to them. If any one of the factors in building blocks 3, 4, 5, and 6 apply to them, then they should seriously consider suspending therapy until they have worked out those particular issues. Failure to do this may cause them physical, psychological, spiritual, or social harm.

The third step is to courageously make the move to do what is right for them. No one can make these decisions for them. In the area of the objective moral order, other persons *have the duty* to try to lead them away from morally wrong procedures because it is *their right* to hear the objective truth. However, subjective realities are personal to them. Other persons can suggest to them certain ways of proceeding if the couple is open to it. Yet the decision remains theirs to make.

Trust, openness, and compassion pave the way in leading the couple to make moral decisions that reflect God's plan for love and life. In terms of compassion, the true meaning of the word becomes evident when its Latin roots are reflected upon. *Cum* means "with" and *passio* means "emotion or suffering." Thus compassion means *with suffering*.

Pastoral workers, in showing compassion, must be willing to suffer with those in their care. If we speak only the "hard word" we will lose them. If we calm their hearts and build a relationship with them, we can take the next step, which is relaying the hard word in love. Yet, once the hard word is related, you must be willing to walk with the couple in their journey to wholeness. If you are not willing to do this, then it is in the best interest of the couple for you to refer them to someone who is willing to speak the truth in love and to spend the necessary time to shepherd them through the healing process.

Conclusion

Certainly we do not wish to ignore the serious difficulties that Christian spouses might encounter, since for them as for everyone, "the gate is narrow, and the way is difficult that leads to life."[17] Nevertheless, their way will be illuminated by the hope of this life as long as they strive courageously "to live wisely and justly and piously in this world,"[18] knowing that "the form of the world passes away."[19].

Therefore, spouses must willingly take up the labors that have been assigned to them, strengthened both by faith and by hope, which "do not disappoint because the charity of God is poured into our hearts through the Holy Spirit who is given to us."[20] They must constantly pray for divine assistance and especially drink of grace and charity from the eternal font of the Eucharist. If they are hampered by sin, they must not lose heart, but humbly and constantly flee to the mercy of God, which the sacrament of penance abundantly provides. It is by this way of life that spouses will be able to advance toward perfection in their married life.[21]

Couples intimately experiencing infertility know the sorrows and difficulty that sometimes accompany married life. In the great scheme of things that can plague a marriage. Infertility is not as severe as substance abuse, domestic violence, or debilitating and life threatening illness, however, it is no less devastating.

How do we care for such couples with compassion and yet remain faithful to the truth which will ultimately raise their dignity and bring them healing? Our first words to them should be **"Do Not Be Afraid!"**

Do Not Be Afraid of God. He has not abandoned you, nor has He left you to face this difficulty on your own. He does not hold things against you. He only asks that you look at your actions in light of the truth and correct that which needs to be corrected.

Do Not Be Afraid of the Church. The Church is your Holy Mother who seeks to gather her children and instruct them in the ways of God. Through her hands God heals and nourishes His children. Christ did not come into the world to condemn it, He came so that all would have abundant life. So too does the Church seek not to condemn but to bring you wholeness.

> The Church cannot abandon man, for His "destiny," that is to say his election, calling, birth and death, salvation or perdition, is so closely and unbreakably linked with Christ…Man in the full truth of his existence…and in the sphere of the whole of mankind—This man is the primary route that the Church must travel in fulfilling her mission: *He is the primary and fundamental way for the Church,* the way traced out by Christ Himself, the way that leads invariably through the mystery of the incarnation and the redemption.[22]

Do Not Be Afraid!

Notes

1. John Paul II, *Familiaris Consortio: The Role of the Christian Family in the Modern World.* (1981), 11.
2. The Pontifical Council for the Family, *The Truth and Meaning of Human Sexuality.* (1995), 10.
3. *Ibid.*
4. John Paul II, *Familiaris Consortio.* (1981), 14.
5. Congregation for the Doctrine of Faith, *Donum Vitae Part II: Instruction on Bioethics: Respect for Human Life.* (1987), 8.
6. A child is not something *owed* to one, but is a *gift.* The "supreme gift of marriage" is a human person. A child may not be considered a piece of property, an idea to which an alleged "right to a child" would lead. In this area, only the child possesses genuine rights: the right "to be the fruit of the specific act of the conjugal love of his parents," and "the right to be respected as a person from the moment of his conception." See Libreria Editrice Vaticana, *Catechism of the Catholic Church* (Washington, DC: United States Catholic Conference, 1997), 2378.
7. Genesis 1:27-28
8. Genesis 2:7
9. Genesis 2:18
10. John Paul II, *Theology of the Body: Human Love in the Divine Plan.* (Boston, MA: Daughters of St. Paul, 1997).
11. Genesis 2:21-22
12. John Paul II, *Theology of the Body: Human Love in the Divine Plan.*
13. Genesis 2:23
14. Genesis 2:15-17
15. John Paul II, *Veritatis Splendor.* (1993), 35.
16. Pope Paul VI, *Gaudium Et Spes: Pastoral Constitution on the Church in the Modern World.* (1965), 50.
17. Matthew 7: 14
18. Titus 2:12
19. 1 Corinthians 7:31
20. Romans 5:5
21. Pope Paul VI, *Humanae Vitae.* (1968), 25.
22. John Paul II, *Redemptor Hominis.* (1979), 14.

Part II:

Science, Philosophy and the Human Being

CHAPTER 5

What's Wrong with Biology and Biologists? The Remote Roots of the Moral Crisis

Daniel P. Toma[1]

In his work, *On the Truths of the Catholic Faith* (*Summa Contra Gentiles*), St. Thomas Aquinas states that a correct understanding of nature is necessary for a correct understanding of both man's place in nature and a correct understanding of religion and the moral precepts that flow from it:

> The consideration of creatures is also necessary to set aside errors, not only for the building up of truth, but also for the destruction of errors. For errors about creatures sometimes lead one astray from the truth of faith, so far as errors are inconsistent with true knowledge of God.... *Through ignorance of the nature of things, and consequently, of his own place in the order of the universe, this rational creature, man, who by faith is led to God as his last end, believes that he is subject to other creatures to which he is in fact superior.* Such is evidently the case with those who subject human wills to the stars.... It is therefore evident that the opinion is false of those who asserted that it made no difference to the truth of faith what anyone holds about creatures, so long as we think rightly about God. *For an error concerning creatures, by subjecting them to causes other than God, spills over into false opinion about God, and takes men's mind away from Him, to whom faith seeks to lead them.*[2]

Therefore, a correct approach to creatures (nature) is so important because while the Catholic faith (revelation) teaches us the ultimate nature of reality and gives us the means to salvation, the understanding of how to think properly about reality (while aided by grace) is not *per se* given by the faith, but is learned by a proper understanding of nature. Revelation and grace are given men not to replace their nature, but to heal, perfect, uplift, and ultimately transform it.[3] Thus, humans know according to the mode of the nature they possess;[4] truths revealed to them do not replace this ability. The nature of man is both soul and body. Being endowed with his senses, he learns first through these senses[5] by studying the nature of things that are accessible to his material being: humans, animals, plants, and non-living things. Of course, his knowledge does not stop at the senses or the imagination, but extends to his reason and intellect.[6] The point to emphasize is that knowledge starts from the senses, which leads to a basic but inescapable belief about creatures. Hence, if humans do not understand the nature of other creatures, they fail to see the distinction between creatures and themselves, thus blurring or destroying what makes humans unique.

Our understanding of our position in universe, and of our relationship to God, is therefore affected. If we have false beliefs about our nature and the natures of things around us, and behave in a manner that is consistent with these falsehoods, we will not act morally, for moral behavior proceeds from nature.[7] We do not expect a dog to behave like a human, for the simple reason that the dog is not a human. If our minds are open to the proper way to approach the study of nature, the nature of creatures teaches us to properly make distinctions about ourselves and the rest of reality.

This position of St. Thomas was recently echoed by Pope John Paul II, in his encyclical letter, *Fides et Ratio*, where he states the Catholic position on the relationship between things known by nature, the material universe, and things known by revelation, as follows:

> ...the God of creation is also the God of salvation history. It is the one and same God who establishes and guarantees the intelligibility and reasonableness of the natural order of things upon which scientists confidently depend, and who reveals himself as the Father of our Lord Jesus Christ.[8]

The Church therefore holds that there is a certain commonality between natural and supernatural beings, and hence natural and supernatural truths. This is based on the truth that God created both orders as a reflection of his being, or as St. Thomas states, God's knowledge of Himself causes things to exist as multiple ways of reflecting His essence.[9] He primarily and essentially knows only Himself and thus knows other things through Himself.[10] Thus, the same principles of being that apply to the material universe apply analogously to revealed things, since they are both "rooted" in the Divine Nature. By extension, these laws apply as well to non-material reality attainable by human reason.

This idea has been traditionally maintained by the Church, being taught, among other places, by the First and Second Vatican Councils, St. Thomas, and Scripture, as well as human reason.[11] So confident is the Church of this commonality between both orders of reality that John Paul II notes She asks the faithful to believe that the existence of God can be known by human reason, "The Council began with the basic criterion, presupposed by revelation itself, of the natural knowability of the existence of God, the beginning and end of all things..."[12] John Paul II sums up this course of thought by stating, "...the two modes of knowledge [philosophy and revelation], lead to truth in all its fullness."[13] Thus humans can know truth from both orders of reality.

In direct contrast to this doctrine we cite Stephan J. Gould of Harvard University in his recent book, *"Rocks of Ages."* Gould, a major scientific writer and evolutionary thinker, states, "I do not see how science and religion could be unified, or even synthesized, under any common scheme of explanation or analysis."[14] Instead, he posits two totally separate approaches to reality that have nothing whatsoever in common. He calls this theory NOMA (non-overlapping magisterium)[15]. Religion deals with morality and values, while science deals with the world of facts (nature):

> Science tries to document the factual character of the natural world, and to develop theories that coordinate and explain these facts. Religion, on the other hand, operates in the equally important, but utterly different, realm of human purposes, meanings, and values.[16]

Gould mantras the idea, "religion for morality, science for factuality," throughout his book.[17] He sums up his beliefs in a statement diametrically opposite that of John Paul II, not only concerning religious beliefs but also regarding any possible certain knowledge of such things, "I am not a believer. I am an agnostic in the wise sense of T. H. Huxley, who coined the word in identifying such open-minded skepticism as the *only rational position because, truly, one cannot know*."[18] According to Gould, not only do religion and nature have nothing in common, but also only skepticism can accord the former, a "reasonable" position.[19]

John Paul II recognizes that this position is not only the dominant position in academic disciplines, but is dominant among the common person as well. He states concerning this philosophical skepticism that, "It is no longer a matter of questions of interest only to certain individuals and groups, but convictions so widespread that *they have become to some extent the common mind.* An example of this is the deep-seated distrust of reason which has surfaced in the recent developments of much of *philosophical research,* to the point where there is talk at times of the end of metaphysics."[20] He further notes that these problems have become particularly manifest in theology,[21] and he summarizes his thoughts on this topic saying, "In brief, there are signs of a widespread distrust of universal and absolute statements."[22] Indeed, this is the common experience of anyone familiar with these questions; people today consider most questions of religion, non-material being, morality, and even many things about material being as mere opinion.

St. Thomas observes that these problems are not merely the result of a difference in religious beliefs, namely one side believing in God, such as John Paul II, and the other not, such as Stephan J. Gould. Rather, their opposition arises from a fundamentally different approach to nature. The position held by John Paul II and St. Thomas proceeds from an approach to nature, which allows the human mind to grasp the scientific truths about nature, in addition to ascending to the existence of non-material being and to the existence of an ultimate being. It provides a rational basis for the sciences, in addition to a rational basis for belief in religion, such as proofs for immaterial being, and rational knowledge for moral truths. Gould on the contrary, proceeds from an approach to nature closed to these realties. Gould's approach, scientific materialism, if you will, is fundamentally flawed in its *ultimate* approach to nature, because as a matter of philosophical principle, it assumes there is no reality accessible to the intellect, based upon our experience of nature, i.e. the material universe. Scientific materialism dogmatically asserts that the only way to get at the truths of nature is to apply the scientific method. Of course, since the scientific method limits itself to the study of matter alone (since it is bound by quantity, or measurement—a material property), matter becomes the only objective reality open to rational investigation.

However, science's materialism can be distinguished from science's *methodological* approach to the study of matter. The scientific method is a marvelously effective and valid way to study nature, but it is not the only way to study nature. Indeed, it is one of two ways to approach the study of nature, and is inherently limited. Scientific materialism is a false philosophy that follows from a dogmatic and hegemonic application of the scientific method. Once again, this is to be distinguished from its *methodological* approach in gathering data and facts about nature, which is sound. Thus, scientific data itself is sound.

Thus, the conflict between religion (and morals) and scientific materialism stems from the prevailing scientific philosophy and not from the scientific method properly understood. The consequent loss of a distinction of humans from other creatures flows from this philosophy and not the methods of science. It is this philosophy of materialism that has resulted in a grave moral crisis facing modern civilization. Many biological techniques, such as abortion, contraception, euthanasia, human cloning, and in-vitro fertilization, which were perfectly acceptable (technology permitting) throughout history for animals in agriculture, are now routinely applied to humans—a reasonable approach if there is truly no difference in kind between humans and animals. Further, as is readily evident to any following these problems, the scientific community is among the principal proponents of these techniques.

Unfortunately, the approach to reality of scientific materialism has been adopted by other disciplines, which, in their desire to be "scientific," have adopted this method of inquiry, which is not suited to the unique nature of their study. Therefore, the scientific approach to nature is no longer specific to the physical sciences, but has become the principal means of understanding nature used by other modern intellectual disciplines. Consequently, scientific materialism has crept into the findings of these disciplines. The seriousness of this cannot be overstated. Even in the Church's loftiest teachings of man's relationship with God, mystical theology, a correct understanding of nature is deemed necessary.[23] By nature, humans can know intellectually. Therefore, faith needs nature (St. Thomas in the first quote above uses the word, *necessary*) in order to teach men to reason correctly, and consequently to think properly about the Faith. In other words, revelation, by itself, is *insufficient* to teach men to think, and is therefore *dependent*, in a way, upon nature. This is because revelation, while not arising from human nature, presupposes it, since it is given and expressed according to a human mode of understanding.[24]

Therefore, it is proposed that the present philosophical approach taken by science, not only is flawed, but also is fundamentally incompatible with both human reason and the Catholic faith, and precludes any truly meaningful dialogue between science and the Faith.

What, therefore, is the correct approach to nature which can lead to the position of John Paul II and the Catholic faith, and how does this differ from the approach used by science? *When asking what is the correct, or true approach, the first thing to be asked is not what is true or false, but what is most knowable and least knowable. For a judgment of truth or falsity is made about something, and not in a vacuum. Thus, the first step in any inquiry is to determine what is known and not known.* To understand how this is determined regarding nature, one can cite arguably the two most insightful paragraphs in all of philosophy. In the *Physics*, Aristotle states:

> When the objects of an inquiry, in any department, have principles, causes or elements, it is through acquaintance with these that knowledge and understanding is attained. For we do not think we know a thing until we are acquainted with its primary causes or first principles, and have carried our analysis as far as its elements. Plainly, therefore, in the science of nature too our first task will be to determine what relates to its principles.
>
> The natural way of doing this is to start from the things which are more knowable and clear to us and proceed towards those which are clearer and more knowable by nature; for the same things are not knowable relatively to us and knowable without qualification. So we must follow this method and advance from what is more obscure by nature, but clearer to us, towards what is more clear and more knowable by nature.[25]

What does Aristotle mean by this? Implicitly at least, these two paragraphs are agreed to by every man, woman, and child. For it does not outline an opinion, but states the mode by which humans come to know and discover things.[26] Every sentence, paragraph, and process with which we communicate knowledge proceeds as Aristotle has described.

Therefore, using the first sentence of the second paragraph as a point of explanation, one can explain this by the use of a rather simple occurrence that most people have experienced, that of tasting food another person has never tasted. When this occurs, and the second person asks the question, "What does it taste like?" they are asking to have the unknown food related to one familiar to them. In other words, they come to understand the unfamiliar based on what is more known. This occurs in many common human experiences, such as the same question applied to an unfamiliar place, "What was the place like?" or an unfamiliar person, "Who was he/she like?" In all these cases, the unknown is explained on the basis of the known. Verbs are another simple example. Most verbs describe common everyday experiences and are extended to things less known. In the statement, "electricity flows through the wires," "flows" is a verb taken from the common experience of water; no one has ever seen electricity flow, and in point of fact it may not actually flow like water. However, we can only describe things based on what we know.

A more technical illustration can be used in the form of an aeronautical engineer and aeronautical engineering. Aeronautical engineering is based upon several principles, two of which are Bernoulli's' principle[27] and the laws of gravity.[28] The laws of gravity describe mathematically the force exerted by an object's mass in drawing another object to itself. Bernoulli's principle describes how the differential flow of air over a plane wing causes a region of lower pressure on the top of the wing relative to the underneath. This, in turn, causes the plane to be drawn or lifted up into the air. Neither of these two principles was proven by aeronautical engineering, but both were known to be true, or proven, by physics. The aeronautical engineer thus knows them as true at the beginning of his craft. Upon these two principles the design of the aircraft is guided. The wings, fuselage, and tail are all designed to maximize the effect of Bernoulli's principle to offset the most apparent effect of gravity, which is to make things heavier than air fall that are not already in contact with the ground. Thus the plane is designed, or "known" as a device to utilize Bernoulli's principle to overcome this first effect of gravity. In addition, no success or failure in the design of the aircraft will affect the validity of Bernoulli's principle or the law of gravity. For example, if the aircraft would not fly, it would be ludicrous to claim that laws of gravity were not valid.

Going one-step back, Bernoulli's principle and the laws of gravity, as mentioned, are known from physics. Focusing on the initial formulation of the laws of gravity, the "given," or the premise, at the beginning of inquiry is the simple observation of gravity - dense objects falling toward earth, such as Newton's apple. Like Bernoulli's principle with the aircraft, the simple observation of gravity was the most known thing and guided and defined the conclusions. For if Newton would have devised a mathematical statement showing objects went up, he would have known it to be wrong. The simple observation of objects falling kept his formulation in line with reality. The actual event was not doubted. However, no amount of success or failure on the part of Newton would have increased or decreased the certitude of the simple observation of gravity.

In education too, this order described by Aristotle is followed. If a child wants to know what gray is, one does not shield from their view all instances of black and white. Gray is defined as a greater or lesser participation in black and white; gray is known on the basis of black and white. Also, there are shades of gray which one may never be able to estimate whether are more black or white. This, however, does not mean one does not know black and white, or color for that matter.

Thus the statement, "The natural way of doing this is to start from the things which are more knowable and clear to us and proceed towards those which are clearer and more knowable by nature..." is clarified. This leads to the following two generalizations about knowledge.[29] First, in any given body (process) of knowledge, what is most known are the initial premises. By these premises, the conclusions are found (understood). Second, the conclusions do not affect the knowability of the premises.

In order to clarify this order of knowing stated by Aristotle in the *Physics* and how this pertains to scientific discovery, at least regarding methodology, a few examples will be given. First an example from art will be used, since art is more known to most people than the procedures of science and can be used as a comparison to scientific examples. This will be followed by two examples of how this order of knowing guides scientific research in general, followed by one example of how it guides a specific scientific technique.

First, consider Michelangelo's Pieta and Moses; both are two different statues sculpted out of marble. At the beginning of his work, what was most known (premise) was what he intended on making, the idea of the Pieta or Moses. These ideas guided his process of sculpting. In the Pieta, he wanted to make the sorrowing Mother of God with both grief and love in her face; he placed the curves and lines in her face to show this. In the Moses, he wanted to show in the face of the lawgiver a certain transcendence beyond material reality; therefore the eyes are looking "beyond" the present. Thus, the statues are "known" by the idea. However, even if Michelangelo had not made the statues exactly in the manner he had wanted, this would not have led him to say that he didn't want to make a Pieta or Moses. The conclusions, again, do not affect the original intention. This last point brings up an additional observation, that in the finished product, there is something relative. No one can say with certitude that the finished Pieta or Moses is exactly the way Michelangelo wanted it. He could have made them larger or smaller; he could have cut a given part of the robe of Mary at a slightly different angle, or even excluded certain parts, such as the hand of Christ by covering it with Mary's robe. *How* he wanted to make it is therefore partly relative; *what* he wanted to make is quite obvious from looking at the statue.

The same can be said of an example from science, the human genome project. What was most known at the beginning of the work was the simple fact that one began with a human. To get human DNA, the researcher did not go to a bear, but a human; if you want to learn something about a human you start with a human, which is known before the experiment. The unknown, DNA, is named on the basis of what is more known. We do not say "DNA human," but "human DNA." Likewise we do not say, "genome human," but "human genome." Hence, once again the premises guide the conclusions. No amount of knowledge of the conclusions will affect the simple truth of what we started with, a human. People, who hear the news that the human genome sequencing is done, do not all of a sudden better know that they are human. The conclusions do not change what a thing is. Once again, as with the finished Michelangelos, there is relativity in the conclusions. The estimated number of 32,000 genes in the human genome has changed from time to time[30], and may never be known with certitude. Likewise the number of nucleotides, the building blocks of DNA and the object the sequencing machine reads, is even more relative, as the number can fluctuate between individuals due to such things as allelic variation in genes[31].

The same can be said of red light. People knew the color red long before they knew the wavelength of red. Our ancient ancestors in France drawing cave art 30,000 years ago could recognize red ochre just as well as we can, despite our more detailed knowledge of its composition. When the first scientist who subjected red light to analysis found its wavelength (visible red light to a human) to be 650-700 nm[32], he knew this to be the wavelength of red because he knew he was initially using red light. Further, any piece of scientific equipment can be refined and better calibrated. It may be found in the future that red is 699.999992765, instead of 700 nm. Thus, the conclusions are relative, to a degree.

All knowledge gathered from scientific apparatus follows this procedure as well. For example, one of the most common techniques in a molecular biology lab is running DNA or RNA on an agarose gel[33] to determine the fragment size, a necessary first step in many molecular biological experiments. An agarose gel is made from powdered agarose placed into an aqueous buffer. It is heated to melt the powder, poured into a mold, and solidifies upon cooling. DNA is loaded into wells at one end and ran towards the other by electric current. The larger the DNA fragment, the slower the migration. This occurs because the gel is porous; the larger the molecule of DNA, the harder it is for it to pass through the gel matrix, hence the slower the migration. In addition, a standard consisting of DNA fragments of known size is run parallel to the unknown samples. So here we have two levels of the unknown being determined from the known. First, one concludes to the general fact that a faster DNA molecule (visible as bands on the gel), is smaller because one knows smaller DNA fragments migrate faster on the gel due to the gel matrix. Second, because no two gels are exactly the same (one might not add exactly the same amount of powder, thereby causing slightly different densities from gel to gel), one judges the unknown size, more specifically, by comparison to the standard, which is better known. Even the term "standard" (as that which is more known and other things are judged by) reflects this process of knowing outlined by Aristotle. In conclusion, the unknown DNA size is judged by the standard and the general knowledge of agarose gel properties—properties that cause smaller fragments to move faster. Finally, there is a certain relativity in the conclusions; since it is very hard to judge the exact size of the fragment, one simply states it is "around" a given size.

All these examples lead to the conclusion that what is most known (the initial "given") is more certain than the conclusions, which while more detailed (the finished Pieta or Moses, the number of genes in a human, the wavelength of red light) are less certain and more relative. All our common experiences proceed in this manner. When one cooks, for example, it is very easy to know *what* to make with certitude (just decide what to make). However, the conclusions, or results, are much more uncertain and relative (one might burn them or not get them chewy enough). Hence the very next sentence of Aristotle's, after the first two paragraphs cited above in the *Physics*, "Now what is plain and clear at first is rather confused masses..."[34]

The experience of science is no exception, as we have seen with the examples of aeronautical engineering, the human genome project, red light, and agarose gels. Therefore, the point made earlier in the discussion stating that the methodology and data of science are sound. It *must* follow this order of knowing stated by Aristotle because it is not an opinion, but the universal mode by which humans come to understand the specific causes of things. No less of a scientist than Niels Bohr, one of the two founders of quantum mechanics, understood this when he stated that, "all account of physical experience is, of course, ultimately based on common language, adapted to orientation in our surroundings and tracing of relationships between cause and effect."[35] Every experiment begins with certain conditions and controls one sets up (cause), which produce effects. It would therefore be impossible for science to ever say cause and effect in general did not exist. In effect, it would be stating that the very conditions upon which the experiment was built and the thing that delivered the data (cause and effect) were invalid, a patent contradiction.

However, while scientists follow the method of Aristotle at a methodological level, as shown above, at a theoretical level, they deny it—*since they tend to assume as evident some of science's most important, but still uncertain conclusions.* In its ultimate approach to nature and interpretation of its data, science takes its conclusions and posits them as the premises upon which all of nature is to be understood, similar to the aeronautical engineer claiming, that since he couldn't get the plane to fly, that Bernouli's law had changed. It inverts the whole order of knowing by basing knowledge upon that which is least known and relative, the conclusions. This is the critical problem resulting in the fractionation of modern intellectual pursuits; any possibility of mutual interaction and communication between science and other branches of knowledge, such as philosophy and theology, has been lost, since they all have their mutual connection in the order of knowing outlined in Aristotle's philosophy of nature.

Since this problem has penetrated deeply in many areas of science and non-scientific disciplines, several examples from important areas of scientific research and a non-scientific example will be given. An important point to bear in mind is, once again, the data are not in dispute, but their interpretation according the problem outlined above.

A good place to explicate this inverted order of understanding is in the approach scientists take in educating other scientists, for in education, one conveys knowledge according to manner one knows. The table of contents (paraphrased) of two introductory, undergraduate biology textbooks from major universities illustrates the modern approach as follows:

Part 1: Molecules to Cells 1. Mr. Darwin and the meaning of life: evolution and reduction of life, 2. Small molecules: electrons, atoms, molecules, elements, etc.; Part 2: Molecular Biology and Heredity: Genetics and Gene Regulation; Part 3: Evolution; Parts 4, 5, 6: Microorganisms, Plants, Animals (invertebrates, vertebrates) & their Physiology, Behavior and Ecology[36]

Introduction: Themes in the study of life; Unit 1: Chemistry of Life; Unit 2: The Cell; Unit 3: Genetics; Unit 4: Mechanisms of Evolution; Unit 5: Evolutionary History and Biological Diversity; Unit 6: Plant Form & Function; Unit 7: Animal Form & Function; Unit 8: Ecology[37]

Keeping in mind Aristotle's statement that one proceeds from what is more to the less known, one can see from both examples that this is not what is occurring in biology education. Both texts begin with what is least known and removed from common experience (electrons, atoms, molecules, cells, and evolution), and ends up with what is most known (animals and their behavior). The conclusions of biology and chemistry (atoms, evolution, etc) are the basis upon which one is to understand higher things and those of common experience (macroscopic living things). Biology is the science of life, what it should start with is the distinction between the living and non-living, or even between humans and other life forms, since what a human most knows is himself (yourself is the most known thing to you, because that is what you are). The order of understanding above destroys this distinction, resulting in statements such as, "Despite the advances in knowledge in recent years, for many people the notion of a vital force of some sort still survives. The view taken here is that such a notion is not needed for an understanding of living systems—that all actions and reactions that occur in living systems can be explained in terms of their chemistry."[38]

According to this quote, there is no additional principle of life needed besides complex chemical interactions. This was taken from a graduate-level biochemistry text in a chapter whose title, "The Essence of Living Things,"[39] implies this reductionistic outlook as well. To wit, we can state this problem as such. If you start with the idea that all life is known only through atoms, then the real distinctions between man and monkey, or even, monkey and banana—distinctions which are really quite evident to a six year old—now become much more difficult to understand. At best we are left with differences of degree rather than differences of kind. It is difficult to see what it is about atoms that would give rise to the differences between the man, monkey, and banana. For after all, both man and animal are made of atoms, but looking carefully at atoms one doesn't see a man atom on one side, and a monkey atom on the other! It is only the arrangement of these atoms that vary, and this is not a strong difference, but only one of degree, precisely the point of the philosophical approach of scientific materialism.

This problem is not unique to secular science courses either. The following is a table of contents (paraphrased) from a Christian (used by Catholics and Protestants) homeschooling biology text for grade school:

1. Introduction, 2. Measurement, 3. Collections, 4. Instruments, 5. Seawater: elements, compounds, mixtures, 6. Cells, 7. Simplest cells, 8. Protists, 9. Fungi, 10. Plants, 11. Animals, 12. Nutrition: living chemistry, 13. Disease, 14. Testing for nutrients—more chemistry, 15–22: chapters on physiology, 23 & 24. Plant Growth and Animal behavior, respectively.[40]

Arguably chapter 3 (collections) is where it should be, for it compares different living things of common experience. However, the contents immediately break down according to the previous mode of college-level texts. The structure of this chapter is representative as well of a general problem in Catholic schools. Religion departments are reformed according to orthodox doctrine and teachings of the faith. Also, teachings directly contrary to this in other courses, such as the soul having evolved, are removed. However, the structure of texts outlined above is left in place, which destroys the whole approach to reality and the faith, for as previously stated, we learn to think by correctly understanding nature. What is left in Catholic schools is the doctrine of the faith, and that of science (or a general reductionistic approach to reality in all courses). The result is the NOMA concept (non-overlapping magisterium) of Steven J. Gould, the dominant model of Catholic education today.

Evolution is another concept taught early in both of the cited college biology texts.[41] Once again, evolutionary theory is not readily evident to our senses, but is the conclusion of an extended collection of data over the past 150 years.[42] While it is highly likely that evolution has a role in nature as type of mechanistic causation, it is posited in biology as *the* means upon which all biology is understood, to the exclusion of all other types of causality. As stated by the great biologist Theodosius Dobzhansky, "Nothing in biology makes sense without evolution."[43] However, it is rather evident to our senses that intelligent agents in matter (humans) work through mechanisms to accomplish their ends. Why evolution, according to the dominant thought in biology, disproves teleology or final causality is therefore a mystery.

Perhaps no other scientific discipline has had such a detrimental practical impact on human behavior and morality, based on this "scientific" order of knowing, than psychology.[44] Psychology takes the conclusions of years of research into animal behavior and learning, and aberrant forms of human behavior, and posits them as the principles upon which all of human behavior is to be understood. However, if one follows Aristotle's method, going from what is better known to what is least known, the thing best known to humans is their particular humanity, and then their fellow humans'. If one examines one's self, one must conclude that one has "intentional" consciousness. One is aware of oneself acting as an intentional agent, or a being that acts for an end. If one understands an end, one understands causation, since ends are a type of cause. If one understands causation and ends one can know actions as intrinsically good or bad, and therefore has the freedom to choose good or evil.[45] Hence, one is a moral agent. Modern psychology, even though it studies the development of moral sentiments in children and adults, cannot sustain a claim that human beings are moral agents, because it does not have a doctrine on the intellect. Rather, the repository of morals for modern psychology appears to reside in the emotions. This view contradicts the common experience of humans. This problem is again evident in the following paraphrased table of contents from a psychology text about learning:

> 1. Science and Human Behavior; 2. Pavlovian Conditioning, 3. Operant Conditioning, 4. Pavlovian and Operant Conditioning together, 5. The Stimulus Collage, 6. Behavioral Modification, 7. Primary reinforces and punishers,...15. Thinking, the Self and Self-control.[46]

The least familiar type of learning to a human is Pavlovian and operant conditioning, which have been elucidated by detailed and extended scientific inquiry. Regarding learning, thinking is what is best known to humans. Thus, this approach to psychology educates students based on the things most remote from their senses and experience of reality, exactly the opposite of the approach described by Aristotle. Students, and future scientists, simply take these things on the authority of the textbook author, without making a serious reflection upon their own experience, or by trying to stuff their own experience into the scientific models.

From psychology practiced under this mode of understanding, it can be evidently seen that sciences and morals cannot possibly talk to each other. When each is talking about the human person, they are beginning from completely different starting points, which preclude any common ground for dialog. If as many scientists suggest, man is fundamentally no different than his experimental monkeys, or his lab rats, then only an arbitrary rule, or an emotional sentimentality, will prevent him from experimenting on the man as he would the lab rat. Man is simply a different arrangement of atoms.

Another crucially important example of this inverted order of learning is the recent and widespread scientific inquiry into the nature of consciousness. There is a large effort in the scientific community to equate human intelligence and consciousness with that of animals, or to reduce it to complex material interactions.[47] In other words, this is the same as claiming that human consciousness differs from animals by degree instead of by kind. This is simply the latest assault on the older question of whether or not there exists a hierarchy of being, with some organisms superior to others; the traditional grade going—by increase—from plants to animals to humans. This is a critically important topic for the Catholic faith and humanity in general. According to St. Thomas Aquinas, it is through the intellectual faculty that we know and contact immaterial being.[48] Evidence is cited by scientists in favor of a difference in degree by referring to the ability of animals to do just about anything that humans can do, such as animal communication, structure (nest) building, sophisticated animal societies, and animal learning.[49] Undoubtedly animals do have sense consciousness, since they sense their surroundings, and in many instances quite a bit better than humans.

But, as stated previously, what is best known to humans is themselves as intentional agents.[50] As intentional agents we desire the why, what, what of, and the how of things; we want to know causes.[51] In knowing causes, we are also aware that we can find more than one means of accomplishing a given act. In fact, it is precisely our generalist ability, which indicates our difference in kind from animals.[52] A polar bear is beautiful example of applied material engineering. It can survive one of the harshest environments with relative ease. However, put the bear in the tropics or in space, and it will die of heat or explode. Not so with humans, which can survive all three environments, because they understand the nature and causes of structural and material engineering; hence they can apply it to many circumstances. Animals, not being generalists, do not understand causality.

Now, one might object that they do understand, but simply cannot communicate this to us. This argument, as well, is flawed for the same reason. If animals were intentional agents, it would follow they could find a means of communicating with us. Furthermore, they would want to communicate, since the very definition of an agent understanding cause and effect (wanting to know) implies the desire to do so. Therefore, whatever an animal is, it is not intentionally conscious. It does not know causes and therefore does not know ends, and ends as good or bad. If it doesn't know ends as good or bad, it is not a moral agent knowing right from wrong. Humans, conversely, do know these things and are moral agents. They are, therefore, beings superior to animals or plants. No amount of scientific analysis can contradict this, since this is among the most known things about humans.

As a final example of this problem in the order of knowing, a nonscientific example will be given, since this inversion of the order of knowing is, as previously stated, not peculiar to science. Shown below is a paraphrased table of contents from an introductory textbook on biblical studies.

1. Introducing the Old Testament: What is the Bible, Divine Revelation, and Nature of the Old Testament..., 2. The people and lands of the Old Testament, 3. Archaeology and the Old Testament, 4–25. Chapters concerning literary analysis of the Old Testament.[53]

The structure of this text is reminiscent of the homeschooling biology text. It starts out correct, in part, by stating scripture as divinely revealed, and that it is infallible regarding revealed truths. However, it breaks down into a literary analysis of the Old Testament for the vast majority of the text, setting up the historical-critical method as *the* means to understand scripture. Now what is most known (but not self-evident) in revealed truths are the written tradition of the Church (scripture) and its interpretation and understanding by the oral tradition (the popes, fathers, councils, saints, and doctors of the Church).[54] Therefore, the proper order of learning should be a thorough analysis of the oral tradition of understanding the Old Testament first, and then a discussion at the end, or in another course, of the historical-critical method with its merits and de-merits.[55]

In conclusion, what is wrong with biology, is the same problem for science as a whole and nearly every modern intellectual endeavor to a greater or lesser degree; there is a fundamental error in the ultimate approach towards nature that these disciplines presuppose. It assumes that facts or data, the conclusions of inquiry, are the most known objects of human knowledge. It therefore posits the conclusions, which in truth are the least known and most relative aspect of human knowing, as the premises upon which nature is to be understood. It only follows, therefore, that skepticism is the dominant opinion of modern man, both regarding the common man and the academic. This is the proverbial house built upon sand. More Stephan J. Gould's will arise as a natural course of this education. This has particularly dire ramifications for an understanding of humans and their moral life. When one applies this order of learning to human intelligence and causality via evolution in nature and at a practical level through modern psychology, one destroys the hierarchy of being and the clear distinction of humans from other creatures. It is little wonder abortion, contraception, euthanasia, human cloning, in-vitro fertilization, and Columbine high schools are prevalent in our society - since these actions follow not from an understanding of the uniquely moral nature of the human person, but from self-interest alone. This problem is further exacerbated when the distinction of the living and non-living is removed by reducing life down to the level of chemical interactions.

Philosophy and particularly metaphysics, as noted by the Pope[56] will suffer as well. The great metaphysical proofs for the existence of God and immaterial being are not self-evident, but premised upon the conclusions of natural philosophy, which in turn are derived from the principles of nature found through the method of knowing outlined by Aristotle. While modern man may understand the logical structure of these proofs, they are ultimately vacuous to him, since the absolute necessity of their premises is not understood. Theology, in turn will suffer, once again noted by the Pope[57], since the great Trinitarian, Christological and sacramental (particularly the Eucharistic) dogmas are all stated in terms of classical philosophy. Finally, humans will suffer in general because, as creatures created with intellects, we have an intrinsic right to know the rational basis for religion, our life, and moral behavior. Skepticism cannot satisfy us, and the only way to avoid skepticism is to proceed in our understanding of nature in a manner consistent with that articulated by Aristotle. To quote St. Thomas once more, "From this we evidently gather the following conclusion: whatever arguments are brought forward against the doctrines of the faith are conclusions incorrectly derived from the first and self-evident principles embedded in nature. Such conclusions do not have the force of demonstration; they are arguments that are either probable or sophistical. And so, there exists the possibility to answer them."[58]

The order of knowing outlined by Aristotle is the only one that, in the end, can firmly anchor the sciences and all modern branches of knowing in reality and open to man truths about his own nature, and about spiritual reality beyond nature. It is only through a solid restoration of a philosophy of nature, as understood by Aristotle, and the foundation of scientific and theological education based upon this philosophy of nature, that will make it possible for science and theology to speak to each other.

Notes

1. I would like express my great appreciation to Richard W. Cross for the detailed reading and substantial editing of this manuscript. The author, however, accepts full responsibility for the contents and ideas expressed, and any errors contained therein.

2. St. Thomas Aquinas, *On the Truth of the Catholic Faith (Summa Contra Gentiles)*, trans. Anton C. Pegis (Garden City, New York: Doubleday & Company, 1955), 2.3.1,5,6. Italics added by author for emphasis.

3. United States Catholic Conference, Inc.—Libreria Editrice Vaticana, *Catechism of the Catholic Church*, (Liguori, MO: Liguori Publications, 1994), 1.2. art. 1. Aquinas, In vol. 1 of *Summa Theologica*, trans. Fathers of the English Dominican Province (Westminster, MD: Christian Classics, 1981), 1a.1a. q. 1. art. 1. —. *Summa Contra Gentiles*, 3.147-153, and 4.54-55.

4. Aquinas, In vol. 1 of *Summa Theologica*, 1a.1a. q. 84-89.

5. Aristotle, *Posterior Analytics*, In vol. 1 of *The Collected Works of Aristotle*, ed. Jonathan Barnes (Princeton: Princeton University Press, 1984), 2.19.

6. Aquinas, In vol. 1 of *Summa Theologica*, 1a.1a. q. 79.

7. Aquinas, *Summa Contra Gentiles*, 3.2-3.

8. John Paul II, *Fides et Ratio*, Vatican Translation (Boston: Pauline Books and Media, 1998), 34.

9. Aquinas, In vol. 1 of *Summa Theologica*, 1a.1a. q. 14. art. 8.

10. Aquinas, *Summa Contra Gentiles*, 1.48.

11. John Paul II cites the Second Vatican Council as supporting this position in its citation of the First Vatican Council, "There are two orders of knowledge, distinct not only in their point of departure, but also in their object" (John Paul II, *Fides et Ratio*, 53). He further cites the First Vatican Council as stating, "Even if faith is superior to reason there can never be a true divergence between faith and reason, since the same God who reveals the mysteries and bestows the gift of faith has also placed in the human spirit the gift of reason. This God could not deny himself, nor could the truth ever contradict the truth" (Ibid., 53). Regarding St. Thomas one can cite, in addition to the quotes given in the text, many places such as, "...the knowledge of the principles that are known to us naturally are implanted in us by God; for God is the author of our nature. These principles, therefore, are contained by the divine Wisdom. Hence, whatever is opposed to them is opposed to divine Wisdom. That which we hold by faith as divinely revealed, therefore, cannot be contrary to our natural knowledge" (Aquinas, *Summa Contra Gentiles*, 1.7). Scripturally, John Paul II notes Jn. 1:14-16, 18; Acts 17:23; Rom. 1:20; Eph. 4:21; and Col. 1:15-20 (John Paul II, *Fides et Ratio*, 34). Finally, by human reason, he notes the principle of non-contradiction in that two points of truth cannot contradict themselves, even if from separate orders (Ibid., 53).

12. Ibid., 53.

13. Ibid., 34.

14. Stephan J. Gould, *Rocks of Ages* (New York: The Ballantine Publishing Group, 1999), 4.

15. Ibid., 5.

16. Ibid., 4.

17. Ibid., 41.

18. Ibid., 8-9. Italics added by author for emphasis.

19. Ibid., see discussion on pages 1-90. Gould is ambiguous on the knowability of morals. While he maintains very insistently that he has great respect for reli-

gion, stating it and science are equally important, and that one must gain morals from religion, he maintains the position cited in note 17, that it is impossible to know regarding religion. If it is ultimately impossible to know based upon religion, and morals proceed from religion, why, might one ask, should anyone ever truly adhere to any body of moral principles?

20. John Paul II, *Fides et Ratio*, 55.
21. "In theology too, the temptations of other times have reappeared. In some contemporary theologies, for instance, a certain *rationalism* is gaining ground, especially when opinions thought to be philosophically well founded are taken as normative for theological research. This happens particularly when theologians, through lack of philosophical competence, allow themselves to be swayed uncritically by assertions which have become part of parlance and culture but which are poorly grounded in reason. There are also signs of a resurgence of *fideism*, which fails to recognize the importance of rational knowledge and philosophical discourse for the understanding of faith, indeed for the very possibility of belief in God... Other modes of latent fideism appear in the scant consideration accorded to speculative theology, and in disdain for the classical philosophy from which the terms of both the understanding of faith and the actual formulation of dogma have been drawn." (Ibid., 55).
22. Ibid., 56.
23. John of the Cross, the great mystic and doctor of the Church, says in his *Spiritual Canticles*, "On the spiritual road the consideration of creatures is first in the order after the exercise of self-knowledge." Immediately previous to this, he states, "...[the soul] begins to walk along the way of the knowledge and consideration of creatures which leads to the knowledge of her *Beloved*, the Creator" (italics added by author for emphasis). Note that a correct understanding of creatures is not necessary to simply know the Creator, but the Creator as *Beloved*. (St. John of the Cross, Spiritual Canticles, In *The Collected Works of St. John of the Cross*, trans. Kieran Kavanaugh, O.C.D., and Otilio Rodriguez, O.C.D [Washington, D.C: Institute of Carmelite Studies, 1979], stanza 4.1).
24. Aquinas, *Summa Contra Gentiles*, 1.3-8. —. In vol. 1 of *Summa Theologica*, 1a.1a. q. 1. art. 1. From scripture see particularly Jn 1: 14, "The Word became flesh..." and 1 Jn 1: 1-2, where St. John speaks about what was eternal and from the beginning being made to be seen, heard, and touched, i.e. known by human modes.
25. Aristotle, *Physics*, 1.1.184a10-21.
26. Aristotle, *Posterior Analytics*, 1.1
27. Francis W. Sears, Mark W. Zemansky, and Hugh D. Young, *College Physics*, 5th ed. (Reading, MA: Addison-Westley, 1982), 243-248.
28. Ibid., 59-63.
29. Aristotle, *Posterior Analytics*, 1.1.
30. Ben Shouse, "Human Gene Count on the Rise," *Science* 295: 145 (2002).

31. R.A Wallace, G.P. Sanders, and R.J. Ferl, *Biology: the Science of Life*, 3rd ed. (New York: HarperCollins Publishers, 1991), 231.

32. Sears, Zemansky, and Young, *College Physics*, 5th ed., 642.

33. J. Sambrook, E.F. Fritsch, and T. Maniatis, In vol. I of Molecular Cloning, 2nd ed. (Plainview, New York: Cold Spring Harbor Laboratory Press, 1989), 1: 6.3-6.19.

34. Aristotle, Physics, I.1.184a22.

35. Niels Bohr, "Quantum Physics and Biology," *Models and Analogues in Biology: Symposia of the Society for Experimental Biology* 14: 1-5 (1959).

36. Wallace, Sanders, and Ferl, Table of Contents to *Biology: the Science of Life*, 3rd ed.

37. N.A. Campbell, J.P. Riece, and L.G. Mitchell, Table of Contents to *Biology*, 8th ed. (Menlo Park, CA: Addison-Westley Longman, Inc., 1999).

38. Geoffrey Zubay, Introduction to *Biochemistry*, 2nd ed. (New York, New York: MacMillian and Collier MacMillian, 1988).

39. Ibid., Introduction.

40. Michael J. Spear, Table of Contents to *Life Science: All creatures great and small* (Washingtonville, New York, Spear Printing Co., 1995).

41. Wallace, Sanders, and Ferl, Table of Contents to *Biology: the Science of Life*, 3rd ed.

42. Ibid., 12-18, 372-392.

43. Theodosius Dobzhansky, "Nothing in Biology Makes Sense Except in the Light of Evolution," *The American Biology Teacher* 35: 125-129 (1973).

44. The main points of these ideas concerning psychology are credited to the following writings (and lengthy conversations with) of Richard W. Cross.

    Richard W. Cross, "Aquinas on Psychology," *Journal of Psychology and Christianity*, 18 (1): 30-45 (1999).

    "Is psychology a part of philosophy? The problem of induction in empirical research." In *Moral Issues in Psychology: Personalist Contributions to Selected Problems* ed. J.M Dubois (New York: University Press of America, 1996), 129-145.

    "Can Catholics Counsel, The loss of Prudence in Modern Humanist Psychology." *Faith and Reason* 18 (1): 87-111 (1994).

45. Aquinas, *Summa Contra Gentiles*, 2.47-48; 3.2-3.

46. J.D. Baldwin and J.I. Baldwin, Table of Contents to *Behavioral Principles in Everyday Life*, 4th ed. (New Jersey: Prentice Hall, 2001).

47. There are innumerable recent scientific books on the subject of intelligence and consciousness. Two very popular ones that capture the essence of these arguments are: Patricia Smith Churchland, *Toward a Unified Science of the Mind and Brain* (Cambridge, MA: MIT Press, 1986) and Paul M. Churchland, *Matter and Consciousness, A Contemporary Introduction to the Philosophy of Mind* (Cambridge, MA: MIT Press, 1988). Another recent one is *The Astonishing Hypothesis. The Scientific Search for the Soul* by Nobel Laureate Francis

Crick. What is "astonishing," according to Crick about the hypothesis is that, in opposition to the common opinion of the soul as something immaterial, he thinks science can explain the soul purely on the basis of neural interactions in the brain (Francis Crick, *The Astonishing Hypothesis. The Scientific Search for the Soul* [New York: Simon and Schuster, 1994], 3-10).

48. "It is impossible to attain knowledge of the divine and highest causes except through what we can acquire by actualizing our intellectual power; and if we knew nothing about the nature of this power we should know nothing about the nature of the immaterial substances...We cannot master the science of morals unless we know the power of the soul" (Aquinas, *Aristotle's De Anima and the Commentary of St. Thomas Aquinas*, trans. Kenelm Foster, O.P., M.A. and Silvester Humphries, O.P., M.A. [London: Routledge and Kegan Paul LTD, 1951], 1.1.7). "Understanding is an act proper to the soul alone, needing the body...only to provide its object...Whatever operates of itself independently, has also an independent being and subsistence of its own..." (Ibid., 1.2.20, 55).

49. Wallace, Sanders, and Ferl, *Biology: the Science of Life*, 3rd ed., 1093-1131.

50. See note 47.

51. Aristotle, *Physics*, 2.3.

52. Aquinas, *Summa Contra Gentiles*, 2.82.2.

53. Lawrence Boadt, Table of Contents to *Reading the Old Testament, An Introduction* (New York: Paulist Press, 1984).

54. United States Catholic Conference, Inc.—Libreria Editrice Vaticana, *Catechism of the Catholic Church*, 1.2. art. 2-3.

55. See especially, "According to the saying of the Fathers, Sacred Scripture is written principally in the Church's heart rather than in documents and records..." (Ibid., 1.2. art. 3. 113).

56. John Paul II, *Fides et Ratio*, 55.

57. "Other modes of latent fideism appear in the scant consideration accorded to speculative theology, and in disdain for the classical philosophy from which the terms of both the understanding of faith and the actual formulation of dogma have been drawn. My revered predecessor Pope Pius XII warned against such neglect of the philosophical tradition and against abandonment of the traditional terminology" (Ibid., 55).

58. Aquinas, *Summa Contra Gentiles*, 1.7.7.

CHAPTER 6

The Moral Status of Human Embryos

Patrick Lee

Judging from television and major news magazines, one might get the impression that the abortion issue and the controversy about the moral status of human embryos is another example of the "clash" between science and religion. One might get the impression that the problem arises because religious people, or at least conservative religious people, believe that human embryos have spiritual souls, whereas those on the other side adhere strictly to what science establishes.

Well, the actual truth is very different. In fact, the actual truth is almost the exact reverse. While Christians and Jews believe that human beings have spiritual souls, that belief is simply not the issue in the debate about the status of human embryos. Rather, the important point is that human beings have bodies—for it is the pro-abortion side, not the pro-life side, that often implicitly identifies the human person with a pure consciousness, with something other than the bodily self that you and I are. Moreover, while science alone does not settle the issue, science is completely on the side of the pro-life position.

Let me first present the basic pro-life argument succinctly:[1]

1. You and I are intrinsically valuable (in the sense that it makes us subjects of rights).
2. We are intrinsically valuable because of what you and I are. (As a consequence, we are intrinsically valuable from the moment we come to be.)

3. What we are is each a human, physical organism.
4. Human physical organisms come to be at conception. (A biological proposition: Normally a new and distinct human organism is produced by the fusion of a sperm and an oocyte.)[2]
5. Therefore, what is intrinsically valuable (what makes one a subject of rights) comes to be at conception.

Now, those who argue against the personhood of human embryos and fetuses usually deny either step 2 or 3. That is, either they deny that we are essentially physical organisms, or they deny that we are valuable in virtue of what we are.

So, I will consider in detail these points, and then focus on an objection that has become recently popular in the context of the debates about stem cell research and cloning.

First is the denial of Step 3. Perhaps the most popular argument to deny the intrinsic value of human embryos is the "no-person argument." According to this argument, the human embryo or fetus is a human being, a human organism, but it is not a *person*. The argument is that only persons deserve moral respect; that is, only persons are intrinsically worthwhile, are the sorts of things we should not kill, are entities whose interests we should take into account. But, human embryos or fetuses, according to this argument, are not persons.

Sometimes it is argued that human embryos are not persons because human embryos do not have higher mental functions. Mary Anne Warren, for example, argued that in order to be a person, an entity must have consciousness, self-motivated activity, the capacity to communicate an indefinite variety of types of messages, or the presence of self-concepts.[3] Michael Tooley argued that in order to be a person, an entity must have self-consciousness in the sense of having a concept of oneself as a continuing subject of experiences.[4] They concluded that human embryos have none of these mental functions, proving that human embryos are not persons.

Such arguments of course have some plausibility. It seems obvious that it is morally permissible to kill some things (such as lettuce and vicious dogs) but not others. Where does one draw the line between those things that are permissible to destroy or kill, and those that are not? A long tradition says that the line should be drawn at *persons*. But, what is a person, if not a thing possessing self-consciousness, rationality, and the ability to consciously direct his own life?

However, this argument is gravely mistaken. It implicitly identifies the human person with a consciousness that uses or inhabits a body, whereas in fact we human persons are particular kinds of physical organisms. Their argument is that, yes, the human organism comes to be at conception, but you and I, the human person, comes to be only much later, say, when something with self-consciousness appears. But, if this human organism came to be at one time, and *I* came to be at a later time, it follows that I am one thing and this human organism is another thing.

Such a dualist view of the human person is mistaken. First, I think that we have, at least on one level, an immediate awareness of the truth that we are living bodies. When I take a shower I say that I am washing *myself.* If you strike my face I do not say, "You hit my body," but "Why did you hit *me?*" If while walking past a vase on a coffee table I accidentally knock it to the floor and it shatters, I do not say, "My body did that," but, "I am so sorry, *I* accidentally broke your vase."

Second, we can see that you and I are physical organisms by examining the kinds of actions that must be attributed to us. A living thing that performs bodily actions is an organism, a bodily entity. But, it is clear in the case of the human individual that *it* is the same thing that perceives, walks, and talks (which are bodily actions), and that understands and makes choices (what everyone, including anyone who denies he is a bodily entity, refers to as "I"). But, it must be the same thing that perceives these words on a page, for example, and understands them. Thus, what each of us refers to as "I" is identically the physical organism which is the subject of both bodily actions such as perceiving, walking, and so on, and of nonphysical actions, such as understanding and choosing. The thing that I am, and the thing that you are—what you and I refer to by the personal pronouns "you" and "I"— is in each case a human, physical organism (but also with nonphysical capacities).[5] Therefore, since you and I are essentially physical organisms, then it follows that *we* came to be at conception, and that at one time *we* were embryos, then fetuses, then infants, and so on.

So, what should we mean by the word "person"? A person is a subject with the natural capacity to reason and make free choices. But, that subject, in the case of human beings, is identical with the human organism. Therefore, that subject comes to be when the organism comes to be, even though it will take her several months to actualize the natural capacities to reason and make free choices, natural capacities which are already present.

A second attempt to deny the intrinsic value of human embryos is to deny Step 2 in the argument I gave above. This argument concedes that you and I were once human embryos, and so proponents of this view do not identify the self or the person with a non-physical consciousness. What they say is that "person" is an accidental attribute. That is, it is similar to a "basketball player." Just as you come to be at one time, but become a basketball player only much later, so, they say, you and I came to be when these physical organisms came to be, but we became persons only at some time later.[6] Thus, unlike the first objectors, they admit that you and I once existed in our mothers' wombs. They admit that the thing referred to by "I" or "you" is a physical organism. What they deny is that this entity was intrinsically valuable at every stage of its duration. According to Tooley's view, I am not the same entity as the physical organism that once existed in my mother's womb. Instead, Tooley argues that one thing came to be at conception, and a distinct thing came to be much later. But, according to Thomson, Dworkin, and others, you and I did come to be in our mothers' wombs, but we became intrinsically valuable only at a later time. We could express the difference between the two positions this way: The first objection disagrees with the pro-life position on an ontological issue, that is, on what kind of thing the unborn human embryo or fetus is. This second objection disagrees with the pro-life position on an evaluative or ethical position.

My reply is as follows. Obviously, proponents of this view cannot maintain that the accidental attribute required to be intrinsically valuable (additional to being a human individual) is an *act* or an *actual* behavior. They of course do not wish to exclude from personhood people who are asleep or in reversible comas. So, the additional attribute has to be a capacity or potentiality of some sort. Thus, sleeping or reversibly comatose human beings are persons because they have the potentiality or capacity for higher mental functions.

But, there is a sense in which human embryos and fetuses also have a capacity or potentiality for such mental functions as soon as they come to be. Human embryos and fetuses cannot of course *immediately* perform such acts. Still, they are related to such acts differently than say a canine or feline embryo. They are members of a natural kind—a biological species—whose members, if not prevented by extrinsic causes, in due course develop the immediately exercisable capacity for mental functions. The fact that they develop these capacities shows that members of this species possess, with whatever it takes to develop them, an immediately exercisable capacity, and that only the adverse effects of other causes on them will prevent it. Thus, from the moment they come to be, they have within themselves—given a suitable environment and nutrition—the internal resources necessary to actively develop themselves to the point where they will perform such acts.[7]

So, we must distinguish two sorts of capacity or potentiality for mental functions that a substantial entity might possess: first, an immediately exercisable capacity, that is, one that the entity will immediately perform in response to a stimulus;[8] second, a capacity to develop oneself to the point where one does perform such actions.[9] But, on what basis can one require the first sort of potentiality—as do proponents of this second objection—which is an accidental attribute, and not just the second, which is possessed as part of what one is?

There are, at least, two reasons against such a requirement. First, the difference between these two types of potentiality is merely a difference between stages along a continuum. That is, the real difference between the first and second types of potentiality is a matter of degree rather than of kind. Between the embryo's natural capacities and the developed actualization of these same capacities in that being's adult life there is only a difference of degree, a difference of more and less along the same line. The capacity for reasoning and making free choices is gradually developed, or brought towards maturation, through gestation, childhood, adolescence, and so on. But, the difference between a person and a non-person, or that which has value as a subject of rights and that which does not, cannot consist only in the fact that, while both have some feature, one has more of it than the other. No one should seriously claim that a mere quantitative difference (having more or less of the same feature, such as the development of a natural capacity) could by itself be the basis for why we should treat different entities in radically different ways.[10] Between the ovum and the approaching thousands of sperm on the one hand and the embryonic human being on the other hand, there *is* a clear difference of kind. However, between the embryonic human being and that same human being at any stage of her maturation, there is only a difference of degree.

A second reason against holding that personhood is an accidental attribute, or grounded in an accidental attribute, is as follows. Being a certain kind of thing is an either/or matter—a thing either is or is not an elm tree, a horse, or a human being. But the accidental qualities that could be proposed as criteria for personhood come in varying and continuous degrees. For example, there is an infinite number of degrees in the developed abilities and dispositions of a person's self-consciousness and intelligence. So, if persons were valuable as subjects of rights only because of such accidental qualities, and not in virtue of the kind of things they are, then, since such qualities come in varying degrees, basics rights would be possessed by human beings in varying degrees. If what makes one intrinsically valuable is some degree of F, then having more F will make one more valuable. The proposition that all human beings have equal rights would be simply an arcane myth, to be cast aside as outmoded superstition. For example, if developed self-consciousness bestowed rights, then, since some people are more self-conscious than others (that is, have developed that capacity to a greater extent than others), some people would be "more equal" than others. This would follow no matter which of the accidental qualities proposed as qualifying for personhood were selected. Will proponents of this view agree with Joseph Fletcher, who years ago argued that human individuals with an Intelligence Quotient below 20, or perhaps also those with an IQ below 40, should not be treated as persons?[11] But, if they will not agree, *why* not? Can they give any principled reason for their disagreement? And can they give any principled reason for disagreement with someone who might say that the cut-off point should be 50, or 60, or 70? Clearly, they cannot. Their proposed criterion is an arbitrarily selected degree of development of a capacity that all human beings possess, from conception until their death as physical organisms.

Finally, a third attempt to deny the intrinsic value of human embryos has gained popularity more recently in discussions about stem cell research and cloning. Some have argued that human embryos are not even complete human organisms. It has been argued that cloning shows that each of our somatic cells—for example, a skin cell—has the potentiality, given the right circumstances, of developing into a mature adult human being. But, if that is true, so the argument goes, then that means that one cannot argue that human embryos are persons on the ground that they have the same kind of potentiality. As Australian bioethicist Julain Savulescu said, "If all our cells could be persons, then we cannot appeal to the fact that an embryo could be a person to justify the special treatment we give it."[12]

To reply, I must first point out that the biological evidence supporting the fact that a new organism of the relevant mammalian species is generated with the completion of the fertilization process is overwhelming. When conception occurs normally (that is, in vivo) a sex cell of the father, a sperm, unites with a sex cell of the mother, an ovum. Within the chromosomes of these sex cells are the DNA molecules, which constitute the information that will guide the development of the new individual resulting from the fusion of the sperm and the ovum. When fertilization occurs, a sperm unites with an ovum, and the twenty-three chromosomes of the sperm unite with the twenty-three chromosomes of the ovum. A new cell is produced, which is genetically distinct from the cells either of the mother or of the father. This genetic distinction and the fact that it organizes its growth from within shows that it is a *distinct individual*. The sort of genetic make-up it has and the direction of its growth also shows that it is *human*. But, most important, there is clear evidence that it is a *complete* human being, rather than a functional part (such as a colony of human cells or a beating heart outside the body). In themselves, parts do not have the ability to develop into the mature stage of the whole organism. But, the embryo or fetus, with nothing more added to it than a suitable environment, regularly and predictably matures to the next more developed stage of maturation for a member of its species.

Now, the argument that the human embryo is equivalent to any somatic cell is plainly fallacious. The proposed analogy is false, for two reasons. First, the kind of potentiality possessed by each of our cells profoundly differs from the potentiality of the human embryo. In the case of somatic cells, each has a potentiality only in the sense that something can be done to it so that its constituents (its DNA molecules) enter into a distinct whole human organism (which is a person). In the case of the human embryo, she already has the potential to *actively develop herself* into a mature form of the kind of organism that she already is.

True, the whole genetic code is present in each somatic cell (since each cell becomes specialized, as muscle, skin, etc., by most of that code being turned *off*), and this code can be used for guidance in the growth of a new entire organism. But, this point does nothing to show that its potentiality is the same as that of a human embryo. In cloning, the nucleus of an ovum is removed and a somatic cell is placed in the remainder of the ovum and given an electrical stimulus. Such acts do much more than bring out the latent potentialities of a cell or merely place a cell in a new environment. The somatic cell is unable to produce a new embryo by itself. Instead, it must work together with an enucleated ovum. Unlike a new embryo, it needs more than just the right environment to develop into the mature stage of a human being. A change in environment is merely external; but the result of cloning is an entirely new organism. There is an internal change in the kind of thing present.

The evidence for this is the entirely new direction of its activities and reactions. Thus, the relevant potentiality of somatic cells is merely that their genetic materials can be used, in conjunction with an enucleated ovum, to generate an embryonic human being. But the potentiality of the human embryo, like that of the human infant, is precisely the potentiality to *mature* as the kind of being that it already is—a *human* being. In the context of cloning, somatic cells are analogous to gametes (i.e. sperm and egg), not embryos. Just as a person who comes into being as a result of the union of gametes was never a sperm or an egg, a person who is brought into being by a process of cloning was never a somatic cell. But, you and I were once embryos, just as we were once fetuses, infants, and adolescents. These are merely stages in the development of the enduring organism—the human being.

Proponents of this position seem to think that the pro-life argument that human embryos are whole human beings is simply that they must be, because the human embryo has a complete human genetic code in each of his or her cells. However, that is only *part* of the argument showing that she is a distinct human being. There is other evidence to complete the argument. The other evidence is that the human embryo's genetic code is distinct from that of the mother, the human embryo is growing and developing by virtue of the embryo's own direction, and the direction of this growth is the mature stage of a human being. In other words, having the entire human genetic code shows that an entity is *human*, but other facts show that the human embryo is *distinct* (distinct from any cell of its mother or father). And still other facts show that it is *whole*—not functionally a part of a larger organism, but rather, a self-integrating member of the human species.

The second reason why the analogy between somatic cells and human embryos is false is that it ignores the most obvious difference between any of our cells and a living human embryo, a difference that is crucial for discerning how they should be treated. Each of our cells is a mere part of a larger organism, but the embryo is herself a complete, though immature, organism. Embryonic human beings are distinct, self-integrating organisms capable of directing their own maturation as members of the human species. Somatic cells, in contrast, are not.

The human embryo and the somatic cell are similar in one respect. Each has the entire human genetic code, which *could* in the right circumstances guide the self-development of a whole human organism to maturity. But, the discontinuity is undeniable. The human embryo is actively making use of that genetic information for her own maturation. What proponents of this argument actually ask us to believe is that each of our cells, even while it is part of us and functions as part of the whole organism that we are, is the same kind of thing with the same kind of potentiality as a whole human embryo who directs her own integral organic functioning and actively developing herself to maturity. If that were so, then each of our cells would already *be* a whole organism, only waiting for the proper environment to begin maturation. But, that is absurd.

Scientists, science writers, philosophers, and others involved in debates about how to treat or use human embryos hold various views of the ethics of embryo destruction. The facts of science, however, are clear. Human embryos are not mere clumps of cells, but are living, distinct human organisms. They are the same as you and I in the earlier stages of our lives. With the fusion of sperm and ovum, or with the coming to be of a distinct and complete (though immature) human organism either by (identical) twinning or by cloning, there is present a distinct organism which will (unless prevented) actively develop herself to a more mature stage as a member of the human species. This new organism directs her own growth, coordinating from within all of her elements and forces toward her own survival and maturation.

In sum,

(1) What we are is each a human, physical organism.
(2) We are intrinsically worthwhile because of what we are, not just because of characteristics we acquire at some point in our life.
(3) Therefore, from the moment that human organisms come to be, which is at fertilization, or twinning, or should it occur in the future, cloning—there exists a being with the same kind of rights as you and me.

Notes

1. For a more extended treatment, see my, *Abortion and Unborn Human Life*, (Washington, D.C.: Catholic University of America Press, 1996).
2. See my *Abortion and Unborn Human Life*, Chapter 3. In identical twinning a second human organism is generated with the splitting off of part of the original embryo, though we may not be able to tell which embryo was the original. If humans are ever cloned, a new human organism will be generated with the fusion, and activation (partly by electrical stimulus) of the nucleus of a somatic cell and the cytoplasm of an ovum.
3. Mary Ann Warren, "On the Moral and Legal Status of Abortion," in Joel Feinberg, *The Problem of Abortion,* 2d ed. (Belmont, Cal: Wadsworth, 1984), 102-119. Essentially the same position is taken by Jane English in "Abortion and the Concept of a Person," in Feinberg, op. cit., 151-160.
4. Michael Tooley, *Abortion and Infanticide* (New York: Oxford, 1983)
5. See my "Human Beings are Animals," in Robert George, ed., *Natural Law and Moral Inquiry: Ethics, Metaphysics, and Politics in the Work of Germain Grisez* (Washington, D.C.: Georgetown University Press, 1998), 135-151; Eric T. Olson, *The Human Animal, Personal Identity Without Psychology* (New York: Oxford University Press, 1997), Ch. 5.

6. Judith Thomson, "Abortion," *Boston Review*, 1998, which can be obtained on the Internet at bostonreview.mit.edu/BR20.3/thomson.html. See also Ronald Dworkin, *Life's Dominion, An Argument About Abortion, Euthanasia, and Individual Freedom* (Random House: New York, 1993), 22ff.

7. When speaking about a specification of a basic potentiality, that is, an ability or disposition, we recognize that one can have an ability and yet require intermediate steps to actualize it. If one asks, "Does Jane have the potentiality (or capacity) to run a marathon?" it is perfectly accurate to reply, "Yes, after some training she will not doubt succeed." And the point of the reply is that she is now in that sort of condition—she has within herself the positive reality needed to get to that more proximate readiness. And so it is with the human embryo or fetus. Because of the kind of things they are, human embryos and fetuses have the basic active potentiality to reason; but to actualize that potentiality they must first grow, develop (or develop further) a complex brain, and acquire a certain fund of perceptual experience.

8. Cf. Bonnie Steinbock, *Life Before Birth: The Moral and Legal Status of Embryos and Fetuses* (New York: Oxford University, 1992).

9. Michael Tooley makes a similar distinction, calling the first type of ability a "capacity," and the second type a mere "potentiality." See *Abortion and Infanticide*, 149.

10. Someone might claim that having interests is not a matter of degree but is on the contrary a nonarbitrary line. But by "interest" those who deny that embryos are persons could not mean every tendency in a being toward a fulfilled state, since all living beings have interests in that sense. So, they would have to mean a *conscious* tendency, that is, a desire. Yet, as I pointed out above, it would have to be not an actual desire but the capacity for a desire. But then such capacities will be in the same boat as a capacity for any mental function, that is, there will be varying degrees of it. In other words, what I say above about capacities for mental functions in general will apply to interests as well.

11. Joseph Fletcher, "Indicators of Humanhood: A Tentative Profile of Man," *Hastings Center Report* 2 (November, 1972), p. 1.

12. Cited by Ronald Bailey, "Are Stem Cells Babies?" in *Reason Magazine Online*, at: http://reason.com/rb/rb071101.shtml

CHAPTER 7

Begetting vs. Making Babies

William E. May

Introduction

In October 1999, fashion designer Ron Harris's website, *www.ronsangels.com*, caught national and international attention. On it he set up an auction of the eggs of six superstar models—portrayed in erotically seductive fashion. The bids started at $15,000 to $150,000 for each egg, plus a 20 percent commission for Harris. In the first few days following the news of this story on national television on October 25, 1999, Harris's website had 5 million visits, and Harris then decided to expand the website, adding more supermodels, including men whose sperm would be auctioned off. Three years later (January, 2002) the website (pornographic in nature) boasts that it is "the most visited egg and sperm site in the world," and that "over 5,000 articles and 500 television stations worldwide have featured Ron's Angels."

I have chosen to begin this paper by referring to Ron's Angels website and its wares to illustrate some of the more extreme and grotesquely commercial uses to which the "new reproductive technologies" have led. I acknowledge that these technologies—*in vitro* fertilization with embryo transfer whether homologous or heterologous, artificial insemination whether by husband or vendor, cloning, etc.—were primarily developed to help married couples, unable to conceive children through normal marital intercourse, to have "a child of their own," and we are all familiar with the pictures of a radiantly happy couple holding in their arms the "miracle child" made possible by these new technologies. Without them these couples would still be childless, their homes empty of the joy that children can bring, their hearts aching for a child to whom they can give a home, affection, and love. The fact that these technologies can be put to bad uses in no way shows that their use is necessarily evil. Indeed, the Scriptures tell us that "by their fruits you shall know them," and on the whole the "fruits" of the new reproductive technologies seem to be happy husbands and wives delighting in the love and care they can now bestow on a child who otherwise would not even exist and children whose parents so deeply love them that they overcame tremendous obstacles, endured heavy financial burdens, and patiently suffered (particularly the mothers) the ministrations of medical experts in order to have the child they so ardently desire.

It nonetheless remains the case that these "miracle children" have been generated, not through the conjugal act that makes husband and wife one flesh, but rather through the "new reproductive technologies." That is, these babies are not "begotten" in the act of conjugal love "proper and exclusive to spouses," but are rather the "products" of reproductive technologies. They are "made" and not "begotten." Thus the question can and ought to be asked, is there any significant moral difference between "making" and "begetting" babies? To answer this question I propose that we first (1) distinguish between "making" and "doing," second (2) contrast the "begetting" of children outside of marriage with "begetting" them in and through the conjugal or marital act; and third (3) on the art of "making" babies with the help of "reproductive" technologies.

But before doing this, however, I believe it very important to point out that human babies, no matter how generated—whether through the conjugal act, the copulation of fornicators or adulterers, or by the use of the new reproductive technologies—are *persons,* not things. As such, they are equal in personal dignity to those who have generated them. They are priceless, because the ultimate author of their life and being is the all-holy God who wills to give to them a share in his own inner triune life.

The Difference Between "Making" and "Doing"

Long ago Aristotle clearly distinguished between "making" and "doing," and St. Thomas Aquinas, following the "Philosopher," commented on the significance of this difference.[1] In making, the action proceeds from an agent or agents to something in the external world, to a product. Autoworkers, for instance, produce cars, cooks make meals, bakers bake cakes, and so on. Such action is transitive in nature because it passes from the acting subject(s) to an object fashioned by him (or them) and external to them. In making, which is governed by the rules of art, interest centers on the product made—and ordinarily products that do not measure up to standards are discarded; they are at any rate regarded as "defective." Those who produce the product in question may be morally good or morally bad, but our interest in making is in the product, not the producer. If we did not know the identity of the producer, most of us would rather have a delicious pie made by Osama bin Laden than an indigestible concoction made by Pope John Paul II.

In "doing" the action abides in the acting subject(s). The action is immanent and is governed by the requirements of a moral virtue, prudence. If the act done is good, it perfects the agent; if bad, it degrades and dehumanizes him. It must be noted, moreover, that every act of making is also a doing insofar as it is freely chosen, for the choice to make something is something that we "do," and this choice, as self-determining, abides in us. Thus we can ask the question, are there some things that we ought *not* freely choose to make? Ought we, for example, freely choose to "make" babies?

"Begetting" Children through Heterosexual Congress, Marital and Non-Marital

Until the use of artificial insemination in the late 19th century and the development of *in vitro* fertilization, with its various permutations and combinations in the last quarter of the 20th human babies came into existence as the result of the heterosexual genital union of a man and a woman; and even today this is the most common way leading to the generation of human children.

The man and the woman whose genital union results in the generation of the child can be either married or not married. But it is *not* good for a new human life to come into existence through the copulation of nonmarried males and females. It is not good precisely because nonmarried males and females have failed to make themselves *fit*, through their own free choices, to receive this life lovingly, to nourish it humanely, and to educate it in the love and service of God and neighbor.[2]

Indeed, practically all civilized societies, until very recently, rightly regarded it irresponsible for unattached men and women to generate human life through their acts of fornication; and in my opinion it is a sign of a new barbarism that many today assert the "right" of "live-in lovers" and of single men and women to have children, whether the result of their coupling or the "product" of new reproductive technologies. A great majority of children so generated end up in "fatherless families,"[3] and competent studies have shown that one major sociological result of children who grow up without the care of a father who loves them and their mothers is a large number of teenage youth, in particular boys, prone to violence and crime.[4]

Nonmarried individuals do not have the *right* to generate new human life precisely because they are not married. They refuse to give themselves unconditionally to one another and to respect the "goods" or "blessings" of marriage, among which are children and faithful conjugal love. Nor do nonmarried men and women have the "right" to genital sex. They do not have this right because this unique and intimate way of "touching" a human person of the opposite sex is meant to be a sign of a special union between the man and the woman engaging in it. It is meant to unite two persons who have, by their own free choice, made each other unique, irreplaceable, nonsubstitutable, and nondisposable. But acts of fornication in no way unite irreplaceable, nonsubstitutable persons precisely because those engaging in them have refused to make each other irreplaceable and nonsubstitutable. Such genital acts merely *join* two individuals who remain replaceable, substitutable, and disposable.

But married men and women, precisely because they have freely chosen to give themselves irrevocably to one another in marriage, have by doing so made themselves *fit* to generate new human life. They have, by their free and self-determining choice to marry, given themselves the identity of husbands and wives who *can,* together, welcome a child lovingly and give it the home it needs and to which it has a right if it is to take root and grow. Because they have committed themselves to one another and to the "goods" or "blessings" of marriage, they have capacitated themselves to welcome the child lovingly, to nourish it humanely, and to educate it in the love and service of God and neighbor.

Here an analogy may be useful. I do not have the right to diagnose sick people and to prescribe medicines and courses of action to help them. I do not have this right because I have not freely chosen to study medicine and discipline myself so that I can acquire the knowledge and skills needed to do these tasks. But doctors, who have freely chosen to submit themselves to the discipline of studying medicine and of developing the skills necessary to practice it, do have this right. They have freely chosen to make themselves *fit* to do what doctors are supposed to do. Similarly, married men and women have, by freely choosing to marry, made themselves *fit* to do what husbands and wives are supposed to do; and among the things that husbands and wives are supposed to do is to give life to new human persons and to provide them with the home they need.

In addition, married men and women have made themselves *fit* for and *capacitated* themselves to engage in the conjugal act. By giving themselves irrevocably to one another in marriage, they have made each other absolutely irreplaceable and nonsubstitutable in their lives. As the 20th century German Protestant theologian Helmut Thielicke so aptly put the matter: "Not uniqueness establishes the marriage, but the marriage establishes the uniqueness."[5] Thus, the conjugal act truly unites two persons, one male and the other female, who are absolutely irreplaceable and nonsubstitutable *because they are married.* The conjugal act is not simply a genital act between a man and a woman who just "happen" to be married. It is rather, an act that participates in the marital union itself, an act "open:" to the "goods" of marriage, to the communication of a unique kind of love, spousal or conjugal love, and to the gift of new human life. Thus, if the husband, for instance, in choosing to have sex with his wife, refuses to give himself to her in a receiving sort of way[6] but rather seeks simply to use his wife as a mere means of satisfying his sexual urges, he is not, in truth, engaging in the conjugal act, nor would his wife be doing so were she to refuse to receive him in a giving sort of way.[7]

Now when human life comes to be in and through the marital act, it comes, even when ardently desired, as a "gift" crowning the act itself. When husband and wife engage in the marital act, they are "doing" something, that is, engaging in an act open to the communication and fostering of their unique conjugal love (its "unitive" meaning) and open also to receive the gift of new human life from God should the conditions for receiving this gift be present (its "procreative" meaning). When they engage in the marital act, husbands and wives are not "making" anything: they are not "making" love, because love is not a product but is rather the sincere gift of self. Nor, should human life come as a gift crowning their personal union, do they "make" the baby. The new human life that crowns the marital act of husband and wife is surely not treated as if it were a product. The life they beget is not the product of their art but, as the Catholic Bishops of England accurately noted some years ago, is a "gift supervening on and giving permanent embodiment to" the marital act itself.[8] When human life comes to be through the marital act, we can truly say that the spouses are "begetting" or "procreating" new human life. They are not "making" anything. The life they receive is "begotten, not made."

The "Art" of Making Babies by Use of New Reproductive Technologies

But when new human life comes to be as a result of artificial insemination (heterologous or homologous) or by *in vitro* fertilization and its varied combinations and permutations (heterologous or homologous), it is the end product of a series of actions, transitive in nature, undertaken by different persons in order to make a particular product, a human baby. The males and females involved "produce" the gametic materials, which others then use in order to make the final product, the child. In such a procedure, the child "comes into existence, not as a gift supervening on an act expressive of the marital union...but rather in the manner of a product of making (and, typically, as the end product of a process managed and carried out by persons other than his parents)."[9] The new human life is "made," not "begotten."

Precisely because artificial insemination/fertilization, whether heterologous or homologous, is an act of "making," it is standard procedure to over stimulate the woman's ovaries so that several ova can be retrieved and then fertilized with sperm (usually obtained through masturbation), with the result that several new human beings (zygotes at this stage of development) are brought into being. Some of these new human beings are usually then frozen and kept on reserve should initial efforts to achieve implantation and gestation to birth fail. Moreover, it is not uncommon for several embryos to be implanted in the womb to enhance the probability of successful implantation and, should a too large number of embryos successfully implant, to discard the "excess" number of human lives through a procedure some euphemistically call "pregnancy reduction." Moreover, it is common, in practicing *in vitro* fertilization, to monitor the development of the new human life both while it is still outside the womb and afterwards to determine whether or not it suffers from any "defects." Should serious defects be discovered, abortion is frequently recommended. As a form of "making" or "producing," artificial insemination/fertilization, whether homologous or heterologous, leads to the use of these methods, for they simply carry out the logic of manufacturing products: one should use the most efficient, time-saving, and cost-saving methods available to deliver the desired product, and quality controls ought to be put in place to assure that the resulting "product" is in no way "defective."

One readily sees how dehumanizing such "production" of human babies is. Human babies are not to be treated as products inferior to their producers and subject to quality controls; they are persons equal in dignity to their parents.

Many people, both Catholic and non-Catholic, can understand why heterologous insemination/fertilization is not a morally good way to generate human life even if, in some highly unique situations, they might be willing to justify such ways of generating human life. They recognize that when a man and a woman marry, they "give" themselves exclusively to one another and that the "selves" they give are sexual and procreative beings. Just as they violate their marital commitment by attempting, after marriage, to "give" themselves to another in sexual union, so too do they dishonor their marital covenant by freely choosing to exercise their procreative power with someone other than their spouse, the one to whom they have "given themselves," including their procreative power, "forswearing all others." They likewise recognize that heterologous modes of the new reproductive technologies raise very critical and thorny issues regarding the parentage of the children so produced.

But many of these same people, including Catholics and among them some well-known theologians, note that homologous insemination/fertilization does not involve the use of gametic materials from third parties; the child conceived is genetically the child of husband and wife, who are and who will remain its parents. They also point out that homologous insemination/fertilization does not *require* hyperovulating the woman, creating a number of new human beings in the petri dish, freezing some, implanting others, monitoring development with a view to abortion should "defects" be discovered. Nor need there even be, in the use of homologous reproductive technologies, the use of masturbation—a means judged intrinsically immoral by the Church's magisterium—in order to obtain the father's sperm, for there are nonmasturbatory ways of obtaining it (e.g., through the use of a perforated condom). According to them, if these features commonly associated with homologous insemination/fertilization are rejected, then a limited resort by married couples to artificial insemination/fertilization does not necessarily transform the generation of human life from an act of procreation to an act of reproducing. They conclude that in some instances recourse to artificial insemination by the husband or *in vitro* fertilization and embryo transfer is fully legitimate, since it does not seem to violate anyone's rights but to the contrary seems to help a married couple's love blossom into life. They reasonably demand to know what evil is being willed and done? Cannot married couples make good use of modern technologies to overcome their infertility in order to have a child of their own so long as they refuse to consider freezing "spare embryos," or aborting should some "defect" be detected, etc.?

A leading representative of this school of thought, Richard A. McCormick, S.J., argues that spouses who resort to homologous *in vitro* fertilization do not perceive this as the "'manufacture' of a 'product.' Fertilization *happens* when sperm and egg are brought together in a petri dish," but "the technician's 'intervention is a condition for its happening; it is not a cause."[10] Moreover, he continues, "the attitudes of the parents and the technicians can be every bit as reverential and respectful as they would be in the face of human life naturally conceived."[11] In fact, in McCormick's view, and in that of some other writers as well, for instance, Thomas A. Shannon, Lisa Sowle Cahill, and Jean Porter[12], homologous *in vitro* fertilization can be considered as an "extension" of marital intercourse, so that the child generated can still be regarded as the "fruit" of the spouses' love. While it is preferable, if possible, to generate the baby through the marital act, it is, in the cases of concern to us, impossible to do this, and hence their marital act—so these writers claim—can be, as it were, "extended" to embrace *in vitro* fertilization.

Given the concrete situation, any disadvantages inherent in the generation of human lives apart from the marital act, so these authors reason, are clearly counterbalanced by the great good of new human lives and the fulfillment of the desire for children of couples who otherwise would not be able to have them. In such conditions, the argument runs, it is not unrealistic to say that *in vitro* fertilization and embryo transfer is simply a way of "extending" the marital act.

This justification of homologous fertilization is rooted in the proportionalist method of making moral judgments. It claims that one can rightly intend so-called "premoral" or "nonmoral" or "ontic" evils (the "disadvantages" referred to above) in order to attain a proportionately greater good, in this case, helping the couple have a child of their own. But this method of making moral judgments is very flawed and was explicitly repudiated by Pope John Paul II in *Veritatis Splendor*. It comes down to the claim that one can never judge any human action morally evil because of the object freely chosen, but that one can judge an act to be morally good or morally bad only by taking into account its "object," the circumstances in which it is done, and above all the "end" for whose sake it is done. If the end for whose sake it is done is a "proportionately greater good," then the evil one does by choosing this object (e.g., making a baby in petri dish, intentionally killing an innocent person) can be morally justifiable.[13]

In addition, it seems to me that the reasoning advanced by McCormick and others is rhetorical and not realistic. Obviously, those who choose to produce a baby make that choice as a mean to an ulterior end. They may well "intend"—in the sense of their "further" intention—that the baby be received into an authentic child-parent relationship, in which he or she will live in a communion of persons which befits those who share personal dignity. If realized, this intended end for whose sake the choice is made to produce the baby will be good for the baby as well as for the parents. But, even so, and despite McCormick's claim to the contrary, their "present intention," i.e., the choice they are here and now freely making, is precisely "to make a baby"; the baby's initial status is the status of a product. In *in vitro* fertilization the technician does not simply *assist* the marital act (that would be licit) but, as Benedict Ashley, O.P., rightly notes, "*substitutes* for that act of personal relationship and communication one which is like a chemist making a compound or gardener planting a seed. The technician has thus become the principal cause of generation, acting through the instrumental forms of sperm and ovum."[14]

Moreover, the claim that *in vitro* fertilization is an "extension" of the marital act and not a substitution for it is simply contrary to fact. "What is extended," as Ashley also notes, "is not the act of intercourse, but the intention: from an intention to beget a child naturally to getting it by IVF, by artificial insemination, or by help of a surrogate mother."[15] Since the child's initial status is thus, in these procedures, that of a product, its status is subpersonal. Thus, the choice to produce a baby is inevitably the choice to enter into a relationship with the baby, not as an equal, but as a product inferior to its producers. But this initial relationship of those who choose to produce babies with the babies they produce is inconsistent with and so impedes the communion of persons endowed with equal dignity that is appropriate for any interpersonal relationship. It is the choice of a bad means to a good end. Moreover, in producing babies, if the product is defective, a new person comes to be as *unwanted.* Thus, those who choose to produce babies not only choose life for some, but—and can this be realistically doubted—at times quietly dispose at least some of those who are not developing normally.[16]

In my opinion, the reasons advanced here to show that it is not morally right to generate new human life outside the marital act can be summarized in the form of a syllogism, which I offer for consideration. It is the following:

Any act of generating human life that is nonmarital is irresponsible and violates the respect due to human life in its generation.

But artificial insemination, *in vitro* fertilization, and other forms of the laboratory generation of human life, including cloning, are nonmarital.

Therefore, these modes of generating human life are irresponsible and violate the respect due to human life in its generation.

I believe that the minor premise of this syllogism does not require extensive discussion. However, McCormick, commenting on an earlier essay of mine in which I advanced this syllogism, claims that my use of the term "nonmarital" in the minor premise is "impenetrable," because the meaning of a "nonmarital" action is not at all clear.[17] This objection, however, fails to take into account all that I had said in that essay regarding the *marital act*, which is not simply a *genital* act between persons who happen to be married, but is the "one-flesh," bodily, sexual union of husband and wife (an act of coition) participating in or open to the **goods of marriage**.[18]

It is obvious, I believe, that heterologous insemination or fertilization and cloning are "nonmarital." But "nonmarital" too, are homologous artificial insemination/fertilization. Even though married persons have collaborated in them, these procedures nonetheless remain nonmarital because the marital status of the man and woman participating in them is accidental and not essential. Not only are the procedures ones that can in principle be carried out by nonmarried individuals, they are also procedures in which the marital character of those participating in them is, as such, completely irrelevant. What makes husband and wife capable of participating in homologous insemination/fertilization is definitely *not* their marital union and the act (the marital act) that participates in their marital union and is made possible only by virtue of it. To the contrary, they are able to take part in these procedures simply because, like nonmarried men and women, they are producers of gametic cells that other individuals can then use to fabricate new human life. Just as spouses do not generate human life *maritally* when this life (which is *always* good and precious, no matter how engendered) is initiated through an act of spousal abuse, so they do not generate new human life maritally when they simply provide other persons with gametic cells that can be united by those persons' transitive acts.

The foregoing reflections should suffice to clarify the meaning of the minor premise of the syllogism and to establish its truth.

The truth of the major premise is supported by everything that I have said about the intimate bonds uniting marriage, the marital act, and the generation of human life. Those bonds are the indispensable and necessary means for properly respecting human life. They safeguard respect for the irreplaceable goodness of the marital union and for new human life, which needs a home where it can take root and grow—a "home" prepared for it by the unique love of the spouses.

The Basic Theological Reason Why Human Life Ought to Be Given Only in the Marital Act

There is, in my opinion, a very profound theological reason that offers ultimate support for the truth, set forth in the Church's teaching, that new human life ought to be given *only* in and through the marital act—the act proper to and unique to spouses—and not generated by acts of fornication, adultery, spousal abuse, or new "reproductive" technologies.

The reason is this: human life ought "to be begotten, not made." Human life is the life of a human person, a being, inescapably male or female, made in the image and likeness of the all-holy God. A human person, who comes to be when new human life comes into existence, is, as it were, an icon or "word" of God. Human beings are, as it were, the "created words" that the Father's Uncreated Word became and is,[19] precisely to show us how deeply God loves us and to enable us to be, like Him, children of the Father and members of the divine family.

But the Uncreated Word, whose brothers and sisters human persons are called to be, was "begotten, not made." These words were chosen by the Fathers of the Council of Nicea in A.D. 325 to express unequivocally their belief that the eternal and uncreated Word of God the Father is indeed, like the Father, true God. This Word, who personally became true man in Jesus Christ while remaining true God, was not inferior to his Father; he was not a product of the Father's will, a being made by the Father and subordinate in dignity to him. Rather, the Word was one in being with the Father and was hence, like the Father, true God. The Word, the Father's Son, was begotten by an immanent act of personal love.

Similarly, human persons, the "created words" of God, ought, like the Uncreated Word, be "begotten, not made." Like the Uncreated Word, they are one in nature with their parents and are not products inferior to their producers. Their personal dignity is equal to that of their parents, just as the Uncreated Word's personal dignity is equal to the personal dignity of his

Father. That dignity is respected when their life is "begotten" in an act of spousal love. It is not respected when that life is "made," that is, is the end product of a series of transitive actions on the part of different people.

Conclusion

Some may think that the position taken here is cruel and heartless, unconcerned with the anguish experienced by married couples who ardently and legitimately long for a child of their own and must suffer disappointment because of some pathological condition.

I do not believe that this position is cruel, heartless, and unconcerned with the suffering of many married couples. We must bear two things in mind before looking at some possible alternatives made possible by modern medicine. The first is that husbands and wives have no *right* to have a child. They have no right to have a child because a child is not a thing, not a pet, not a toy, but a person of inviolable dignity. Husband and wives have the right to engage in the sort of action inwardly fit to receive new human life—the marital act. But they do not have a right to a child. Their desire to bear and raise children is noble and legitimate, but this desire does not justify any and every means to see to its fulfillment.

The second point to keep in mind is that we must be realistic and recognize that for some reasons it will not be possible for some married couples to beget a child in and through their marital act. If this is the case, then it is necessary to recognize that we must all carry our cross. But we must remember that Jesus is our Simon of Cyrene, and that He will help us bear any cross He may give us.

Notes

1.   Aristotle, *Metaphysics*, Bk. 9, c. 8, 1050a23-1050b1; St. Thomas Aquinas, *In IX Metaphysicorum,* lect. 8, no. 1865; *Summa theologiae*, 1, 4, 2, ad 2; 1, 14, 5, ad 1; 1, 181, 1.
2.   Centuries ago Augustine rightly observed that one of the chief *goods* of marriage is children, who "are to be received lovingly, nourished humanely, and educated religiously," i.e., in the love and service of God and man. See his *De genesi ad literam,* 9, 7 (*PL* 34, 397).

3. On this see, among other sources, the eye opening work of David Blankenhorn, *Fatherless America* (New York: Basic Books, 1995).

4. See, for example, Patrick Fagan, "The Real Root Causes of Violent Crime: The Breakdown of Marriage, Family, and Community," *The Heritage Foundation Backgrounder,* March 17, 1995; text available at *http://www.heritage.org/library/categories/crimelaw/bg1026.html*; and "Congress's Role In Improving Juvenile Delinquency Data," *The Heritage Foundation Backgrounder*, March 10, 2000; text available at http://www.heritage.org/library/ backgrounder/bg/1351es.html.

5. Helmut Thielicke, *The Ethics of Sex* (New York: Harper &Row, 1963), p. 108.

6. On the asymmetrical complementarity of male and female sexuality, with one (the male's) as a "giving in a receiving sort of way" and the other (the female's) as a "receiving in a giving sort of way" see my *Marriage: The Rock on Which the Family Is Built* (San Francisco: Ignatius, 1995), Chapter Two, "Marriage and the Complementarity of Male and Female," and Robert Joyce, *Human Sexual Ecology: A Philosophy and Ethics of Man and Woman* (Washington, D.C.: University Press of America, 1980), Chapter Five.

7. A remarkable passage in Pope Paul VI's Encyclical *Humanae vitae* brings out this important truth. In it he said that everyone will recognize that a conjugal act (and here he using this expression simply to designate a genital act between persons who happen to be married) imposed upon one of the spouses with no consideration of his or her condition or legitimate desires "is not a true act of love" inasmuch as it "opposes what the moral order rightly requires from spouses" (no. 13).

8. Catholic Bishops of England Committee on Bioethical Issues, *In Vitro Fertilization: Morality and Public Policy* (London: Catholic Information Services, 1983), no. 23.

9. Ibid., no. 24.

10. Richard McCormick, S.J., *The Critical Calling: Reflections on Moral Dilemmas Since Vatican II* (Washington, D.C.: Georgetown University Press, 1989), p. 337. The internal citation is from William Daniel, S.J., "*In Vitro* Fertilization: Two Problem Areas," *Australasian Catholic Record* 63 (1986) 27.

11. Ibid., p. 337.

12. See Thomas A. Shannon and Lisa Sowle Cahill, *Religion and Artificial Reproduction: An Inquiry Into the Vatican "Instruction on Respect for Human Life"* (New York: Crossroads, 1988), p. 138; Jean Porter, "Human Need and Natural Law," in *Infertility: A Crossroad of Faith, Medicine, and Technology*, ed. Kevin Wm. Wildes, S.J. (Dordrecht/Boston/London: Kluwer Academic Publishers, 1997), pp. 103-105. It should be noted that Shannon and Cahill, employing an argument proportionalistic in nature—that is, that it can be morally permissible to intend a so-called nonmoral evil (e.g., heterologous generation of human life) should a sufficiently greater nonmoral good be possible (e.g., providing a couple otherwise childless with a child of their own), insinuate

that, if the spouses consent, recourse to third parties for gametes or even to surrogate mothers might not truly violate spousal dignity or unity. See *Artificial Reproduction...*, p. 115.

13. As noted in the text Pope John Paul II repudiates (and rightly so) this proportionalist method of making moral judgments in his encyclical *Veritatis Splendor.* For a critique of proportionalism see my *An Introduction to Moral Theology* (rev. ed.: Huntington, IN: Our Sunday Visitor, 1994), Chapter 3.

14. Benedict Ashley, O.P., "The Chill Factor in Moral Theology," *Linacre Quarterly* 57.4 (1990) 71.

15. Ibid., 72.

16. The argument advanced in the previous paragraphs was set forth originally in an earlier essay I wrote on the laboratory generation of human life, "*Donum Vitae:* Catholic Teaching on Homologous *In Vitro* Fertilization," in *Infertility: A Crossroad of Faith, Medicine, and Technology*, pp. 73-92, esp. pp. 81-87, making use, too, of material developed by Germain Grisez, John Finnis, Joseph Boyle, and William E. May in "'Every Marital Act Ought to Be Open to New Life': Toward a Clearer Understanding," *The Thomist* 52 (1988) 365-426.

17. Richard A. McCormick, "Notes on Moral Theology," *Theological Studies 45* (1984) 102

18. In her essay, "Human Needs and Natural Law" (cf. endnote 45), Jean Porter claims that my argument in support of the teaching of *Donum Vitae* is based on a "Kantian" sexual ethic, one that "gives pride of place to autonomy" (pp. 100-101). She even claims that I "dissent" from Catholic teaching in my analysis of the marital act because of my emphasis on the role played by intention in determining the moral significance of human action. Porter fails to recognize that my analysis, far from being Kantian, is rooted in the Catholic tradition, which stresses the self-determining character of human actions. My analysis, I believe, is rooted also in the understanding of human sexuality and human action set forth by John Paul II.

19. Here it most important to stress that Christian faith proclaims that the Word Incarnate is still a human being. Christian faith rejects Docetism, the doctrine that the Uncreated Word only seemed to become human and ceased appearing human after the resurrection.

Part III:

Politics and Law

CHAPTER 8

Retrospective and Prospective: The Public Policy Debate on Embryo Research

Richard M. Doerflinger

The Catholic Church has been criticized for having strong objections to techniques whose ostensible purpose is to provide children for infertile couples—that is, to produce new human lives. Some people even ask: What could be more "pro-life" than providing children for these couples through reproductive technologies such as *in vitro* fertilization (IVF)?

The history of the public policy debate, however, dramatizes how closely these technologies have been associated with the destruction of developing human life—especially its destruction for research purposes. This association has reached its high point—or, morally, its low point—in current proposals for using human cloning solely to create embryos *in order* to destroy them.

Our tale begins in 1978, with the announced birth of Baby Louise Brown from IVF. Even this first live birth of a "test-tube" baby was, of course, *preceded* by the deaths of many dozens of human embryos used to refine the process. The immediate reaction by the U.S. Department of Health, Education, and Welfare was to name an Ethics Advisory Board to discuss possible federal funding of *research* on IVF and IVF-produced embryos. Federal regulations issued in 1975 said that no such research could proceed unless a board of this kind was to rule on the ethical acceptability of the research.[1]

The Board's conclusion was that some research along these lines was "ethically acceptable"—and then defined this to mean it would be "ethically defensible but still legitimately controverted." The Board declined to make any recommendation on whether such research should actually be funded.[2] Given this ambivalent conclusion, and a wave of public protest against funding embryo research by Catholics and others, the Carter administration decided not to pursue the research. While the issue was revived for discussion in later Congresses and Administrations, most visibly in 1988, this "de facto moratorium" continued into the Clinton administration.

In 1993, however—emboldened by the election of a new President with negative attitudes toward respect for unborn human life—congressional proponents of embryo research slipped one sentence into a reauthorization bill for the National Institutes of Health (NIH), rescinding the federal regulation requiring Ethics Advisory Board review before experiments using IVF embryos could be funded.[3] (This same bill set new federal guidelines for research using fetal tissue from abortion victims, and with that issue attracting most of the pro-life movement's attention, the single line opening the doors to embryo research went almost unnoticed.)

This left the NIH free to appoint an informal Human Embryo Research Panel that was not covered by federal regulations governing ethics advisory boards—hence the panel did not need to have even a pretense of balanced viewpoints. The chairman, Stephen Muller of Johns Hopkins University, announced at the first meeting that the panel's purpose was to recommend which destructive embryo experiments to fund, not to decide whether this should be done at all. He invited any panel member who disagreed to leave and not come back.[4]

Not surprisingly, the Panel ended up recommending a broad array of experiments involving the death of human embryos—those produced by cloning and parthenogenesis as well as by IVF.[5] This included, for the first time, a recommendation that the government fund research requiring the *creation* of new embryos solely for the purpose of research that would destroy them. And in this regard, the Panel was overconfident, for this aspect of its recommendations created enormous controversy.

The Washington Post editorialized that "the creation of human embryos specifically for research that will destroy them is unconscionable."[6] The Chicago Sun-Times called it "grotesque, at best."[7] Even President Clinton decided that this was a step too far, and agreed to fund only research involving so-called "spare" embryos from IVF clinics. The following year, before his plan could be implemented, Congress banned federal funding of research using "spare" embryos as well, through an appropriations rider to the Labor/HHS appropriations bill known as the Dickey amendment. That rider remains in law today.[8]

In 1997 the landscape changed again, with the birth of Dolly, the first sheep cloned from an adult animal's body cell. Her birth was preceded by the death of 276 born and unborn sheep whose production by cloning was less successful—and it was followed by an inconclusive skirmish over the prospect of human cloning. Following a recommendation by the new National Bioethics Advisory Commission, the Clinton administration recommended a moratorium on cloning humans for *reproductive* purposes only. Pro-life members of Congress favored a ban on cloning used to make human embryos for any purpose. Neither approach received enough support to move forward.

In December 1998, the embryo research debate was thrown wide open again, with announcements that researchers had made advances in their ability to grow embryonic stem cells in the laboratory. Supporters in Congress began predicting, irresponsibly but with a great deal of political cleverness, that these cells could cure every major degenerative disease on the face of the earth. They had learned their lesson from the fate of the Human Embryo Research Panel. They could not simply highlight the wonders of the new research findings. Instead, they had to get well-funded and popular "patient groups" on their side by highlighting an aspect of embryo research that, they claimed, would cure their diseases. The NIH had openly discussed such a strategy in 1994 as a political maneuver for winning acceptance and government funds for embryo research generally[9]. However, until there was some new advance using these cells, proponents could not even make their case *seem* plausible. In politics, as opposed to the actual job of curing patients, *seeming plausible* is all that is needed.

A December 1998 hearing before a Senate subcommittee actually reviewed three ways to obtain embryonic stem cells.[10] To recount the list of approaches is to display a disturbing slippery slope toward closer and closer involvement in the destruction of nascent human life:

1. According to Dr. John Gearhart of Johns Hopkins University, cells very similar to embryonic stem cells, called "embryonic germ cells," could be harvested from reproductive tracts at about eight weeks of gestation. The tissue could be obtained after miscarriage or induced abortion, but only the latter was of great interest to the research establishment. Here the researcher would not necessarily be directly involved in de-

stroying fetal life, but would enter the scene after an abortion had been performed by someone else for unrelated reasons. Obtaining the cells for federally funded research, of course, would require a certain amount of government collaboration with the abortion industry.

2. According to Dr. James Thomson of the University of Wisconsin, embryonic stem cells could be harvested by killing so-called "spare" embryos created by IVF at fertility clinics. Here the researcher would directly kill existing embryos for their useful cells, but would generally not be involved in creating them or in deciding which embryos would be destroyed.

3. According to Dr. Michael West of Advanced Cell Technology in Worcester, Massachusetts, one could create new embryos by somatic cell nuclear transfer (cloning) to get a genetic "match" to each particular patient, and then kill these embryos for their stem cells. This allegedly would solve the problem of tissue rejection. It would also make the ongoing creation and destruction of countless human embryos an integral part of medical practice for each individual patient in need of tissue repair. Here there would be no "immortal cell lines" based only on the past destruction of life, but a continuing project of creating genetic twin brothers or sisters for each patient and then killing them to help their original human model survive.

So what could be wrong with all this medical "progress"? Several things. First, of course, is the moral problem: To one degree or another, each of these approaches involves complicity with the destruction of a developing human life. In fact, the way in which the public policy debate has proceeded on these issues demonstrates the reality of a "slippery slope" leading one to closer and closer involvement with such destruction once the first step is taken. Congress began in 1993 with fetal tissue obtained from abortions, swearing that this in no way involved endorsement of the taking of fetal life itself. By 1998, prominent members of Congress were insisting that the lives of "spare" embryos would have to be destroyed precisely for the sake of research using their cells—after all, they said, these embryos may not be dead yet, but they will soon be discarded anyway. And even then, some were proposing (and many more are now endorsing) the idea that embryos should be specially created only to be later destroyed.

You may think that the real debate is over whether we can really speak here of destroying "human life," because people disagree on "when life begins." But the opposite is true. Every major federal advisory group that has defended destructive human embryo research—the Ethics Advisory Board in 1979, the NIH Human Embryo Research Panel in 1994, and President Clinton's National Bioethics Advisory Commission in 1999—has conceded that the early embryo is a developing human life, and has even said that this life deserves some measure of "respect."[11] In every case, however, the advisory group decided that some human lives lack "personhood" and hence are worth less than others. Most importantly, they decided that the "respect" we owe to these human lives is outweighed by the benefits we can hope to gain by disrespecting and destroying them.

The second problem with the proposals for embryo research is that they contradict many legal precedents at both the federal and state level. Since 1975, one-week-old human embryos in the womb have been protected by federal regulations as *human subjects* who must not be harmed in federally funded research.[12] It is very difficult to argue ethically that the same embryo, at exactly the same stage of development, magically becomes mere research material simply because someone has *chosen* for self-serving reasons not to implant that embryo in a womb. Nine states have laws that are far broader, banning all destructive human embryo research whether publicly or privately funded.[13] Some members of Congress, pressing for human embryo research, like Senator Arlen Specter of Pennsylvania, have demanded federal funding of experiments that are a felony in their own home states.

The third problem is public opinion. While polls with vague and euphemistic language can always be produced to show public support for "stem cell research," the fact is that Americans overwhelmingly oppose the idea of destroying human embryos for research. They also strongly oppose the idea of human cloning—and according to some polls, they oppose its use to make human embryos for research just as strongly as they oppose its use to produce liveborn children.[14]

The fourth problem is precisely this matter of clinical benefits, on which proponents rest all their claims as to why we must overcome our feelings of "respect" for developing human life. It is increasingly obvious that embryonic stem cell research is *not* the only way to pursue promising treatments for diabetes, Parkinson's disease, and so on. The evidence is growing that such research may not offer the best route to such treatments even on pragmatic grounds and, in fact, that it may never provide safe and effective treatments at all. At this point, adult stem cells and other alternatives are advancing far more quickly to provide treatments for these conditions—a development thoroughly documented on the Web site *www.stemcell*

research.org created by scientists and physicians who support morally acceptable stem cell research but oppose the destruction of human embryos for research.

Even President Clinton's bioethics advisory commission concluded that "the derivation of stem cells from embryos remaining following infertility treatments is justifiable only if no less morally problematic alternatives are available for advancing the research."[15] As adult stem cells and other non-controversial cell therapies make progress against diabetes, Parkinson's disease, spinal cord injury, severe immune deficiency, corneal damage, sickle cell anemia, various forms of cancer, etc., it is increasingly clear that embryonic stem cell research cannot pass the test its own proponents have established for it.

Yet when a UFO cult and a group of physicians announced plans to attempt human cloning, researchers—and the patient advocacy groups who follow their lead all too blindly—were prepared to repeat all their past claims for the unparalleled promise of embryonic stem cells, with a new twist. Michael West created genetically matched embryos by cloning, to produce tissue that would be compatible with each individual patient. His method was suddenly endorsed by organizations and members of Congress who had denounced the idea of specially creating embryos for research weeks earlier.[16] Now that Congress had to make a decision about banning human cloning, research groups announced that they had earlier neglected to mention this one little fact: Any cloning ban will have to allow cloning of embryos for research, because that practice is essential to realizing the promise of embryonic stem cell research.

This policy switch was so sudden that it seems implausible to attribute it entirely to a slippery slope. Rather, it seems that some groups knew all along where their agenda would most likely take them, and they also knew that public sentiment would not tolerate the idea of specially creating vast numbers of human embryos solely to destroy them for medical research. So, they posited a more restrained policy as a first step, and bided their time. Announcements by groups wanting to pursue cloning for reproductive purposes forced these research teams to announce their further goal a bit sooner than they would have liked.

By this time, the claim that experimental cloning was an essential road to medical progress was running into more and more contrary evidence. It seemed that the problem of tissue rejection, which cloning was supposed to solve, paled in comparison with other serious problems in embryonic stem cells. These cells were indeed versatile and fast-growing, as enthusiasts claimed—so versatile and so fast-growing, in fact, that they showed a persistent tendency to proliferate in all directions and create cancerous tumors when they, or cells derived from them, were injected into animals.[17] This and other emerging problems helped the House of Representatives to place exaggerated claims for embryo research and cloning in some perspective. In July 2001, the House voted by over a hundred-vote margin, 265 to 162, to ban human cloning for any purpose, including medical research.[18]

Even the policy debate on use of "spare" embryos for stem cell research was then interrupted, if not resolved, by President Bush's decision of August 9, 2001. The President decided that federal funds could be used for research only on existing stem cell lines—those already created by destroying human embryos before his decision was announced.[19] In announcing that these existing cell lines would be used to determine the most promising avenues for exploring future treatments, President Bush indicated one problem with his compromise solution: If this federally funded research discovered paths to new treatments that would require the destruction of many more embryos to meet patients' demand, the Bush policy would in fact lead to the future destruction of embryos, if only by private investors. Those investors have been holding back from gambling on the "promise" of embryonic stem cell research in part because the early stages of basic research yield no profits—investments pay off only when the most promising paths for moving into real clinical use have been discovered. The Bush policy would provide federal funds for this most speculative stage of the research, allowing private funds to move in and replace public funds when the most promising avenues are uncovered. Indeed, HHS Secretary Tommy Thompson declared in congressional testimony that this was the real intent of the policy.[20]

Despite some objections to this approach on both sides of the policy spectrum, however, it soon became apparent that neither side could muster enough support in Congress to dislodge the Bush compromise. And so this issue began to fade from public consciousness until, along with almost all other issues, it was forcibly ejected from our consciousness by the terrorist attacks of September 11.

The embryo cloning issue did return to the policy agenda in late November, when Michael West re-entered the debate with an announcement that his company had succeeded in creating human embryos by cloning.[21] As a scientific "advance," this turned out to be much less impressive than West wanted people to think—he was unable to bring any of these embryos past the six-celled stage and so failed to obtain any stem cells from them. Some critics observed that there was no firm evidence verifying that West had managed to produce normal embryonic development at all. Yet his announcement did produce some sense of urgency in the U.S. Senate, which had been neglecting the House-passed bill to ban cloning. Senate Majority Leader Tom Daschle pledged to bring the issue to the Senate floor in February or March of 2002. He later allowed that pledge to lapse.

The Senate now stands at a crossroads in the cloning controversy. The dilemma facing Senators is sometimes expressed as follows: Should we ban only "reproductive" cloning, or "therapeutic" cloning as well? But this misrepresents the real choice to be made.

The House-passed cloning bill, sponsored on the Senate side by Senators Sam Brownback (R-KS) and Mary Landrieu (D-LA), bans the use of somatic cell nuclear transfer (the cloning technique used to make Dolly the sheep) to make human embryos. It does not ban the use of this or any other cloning technique to make DNA or other molecules, cells other than embryos, tissues, plants, or animals other than humans. It is the only genuine ban on human cloning in consideration.[22]

Senators Feinstein (D-CA), Harkin (D-IA), and others have introduced competing bills that they refer to as bans on "reproductive cloning."[23] In fact, the bills do not ban the use of any cloning procedure for *any* purpose. They allow unlimited numbers of human embryos to be created by cloning, and then ban the act of transferring the cloned embryo to a uterus. This sleight-of-hand is designed to create the appearance of a "ban" while really allowing the unfettered use of cloned embryos in research. The result is that once one has created an embryo by cloning, destroying or discarding the embryo is the only legally accepted course of action. The fact is that government will define a class of developing human beings that it is a crime *not* to destroy.[24]

Besides being grossly immoral, the Feinstein and Harkin bills are likely to be woefully inadequate as attempts to ban even cloning for the purpose of live birth. Once cloned embryos can be readily grown in laboratories, it is inevitable that someone will place such an embryo in a woman's womb. After all, embryo transfer is a standard technique used by *in vitro* fertilization clinics all over the country, and there is no reliable way to distinguish a one-week-old cloned embryo from the fertilized variety. Once transfer to the womb is achieved, there is no way to enforce the ban—unless one wants to try putting pregnant women in prison, or pressuring them to have abortions, so one can claim that we have prevented the advent of live-born clones.[25]

As the National Academy of Sciences recognized in its recent report on human cloning, to clone is to create a new organism that is genetically identical to a previously existing organism. In humans, this is done by making a new human organism at its earliest stage of development, the embryo.[26] The question is whether we will ban human cloning, or allow its use to create a new class of human "guinea pigs" for experimentation.

At this writing, the November 2002 congressional elections have resulted in Republican control of the Senate and increased support for a cloning ban. The genuine ban has been re-introduced in the House of Representatives by Congressman Dave Weldon (R-FL), Bart Stupak (D-MI) and over a hundred co-sponsors as H.R. 234; Senators Brownback and Landrieu plan to resubmit a Senate companion bill, while Senators Feinstein et al. have said they will resubmit their bill to authorize human cloning for research purposes.

What does our future look like if we choose one path or the other? If we allow cloning of human embryos for research, I predict the following developments:

First, this agenda will not stop at stem cell research. Already researchers are showing equal interest in creating embryonic clones of patients with various genetically based illnesses so that they can study the early development of the disease. Some are talking about patenting and marketing certain kinds of embryos as "disease models" for other researchers.[27]

Second, it will not stop at the embryonic stage. The temptation will be to push these limits so more advanced tissues and even formed organs can be harvested for transplant. Already one of the federal bills designed to allow experimental cloning, sponsored by Senator Byron Dorgan, would have allowed implantation of cloned embryos in the womb as long as this is not done to produce "a cloned human being" (which in this bill seems to mean a liveborn human being). This bill would allow cloned embryos to be grown in the womb even to late stages of pregnancy, and then aborted for their organs.[28] It is remarkable that so far there are only two successful animal models for "therapeutic cloning," and they both required developing the clone past the embryonic stage—one study used cloned cow fetuses to produce kidney tissue for the cow that had been genetically duplicated; the other required bringing cloned mice to *live birth* so their genetically modified *adult* stem cells could be transplanted into the original mice.[29] Once we can patent and sell cloned embryos, who's to say that there is a magic moment when they *stop* being property?

Third, it will not stop with replication of the same. Rather, cloning is a gateway technology allowing the development and mass implementation of human genetic engineering. Dolly the sheep was created to solve a problem in the development of genetically "superior" sheep. Genetic modification is so inefficient that it is essential to be able to replicate one's rare successes when they do occur. The same will be true of human engineering.[30] And of course, the technology used to make an exactly identical human can easily be adapted to make a human who is "better" in just one characteristic, or in several. Already recent successes in cloning cats has led observers to predict an age of "designer pets" in which desired traits are listed, bought, and manufactured.[31] Princeton biologist Lee Silver goes farther, predicting a future caste system in which those who can afford genetic enhancement (the "GenRich") become increasingly alienated from those who cannot (the "Naturals"), perhaps in the end becoming a different and superior species.[32] From these developments onward, a full-scale "Brave New World" in which humans are designed, bred, "decanted," and dehumanized seems all too near.

And what happens if we manage to ban human cloning? That will be a good thing in itself, and it will also be important as a declaration that society will not go blindly and unwittingly into the post-human future. It means that new alleged technological advances will have to show that they offer real benefits without unacceptable moral costs, instead of simply being endorsed because everything new is "progress." It will give us some breathing space, and the time to sit back and ask ourselves: How did we get to this point? How did we come to the brink of accepting a "reproductive" technology whose only use was to reduce humans to fodder for researchers? Is there something so inherently depersonalized and dehumanizing about the laboratory production of human life that it tempts us to see our fellow humans as mere objects?

If we can ask these questions about cloning and the creation of embryos for research, we may even begin to look at the reproductive technologies that have produced so many "spare" embryos as possible research material over the last two decades. We may ask whether our society's first wrong turn was in seeing *in vitro* fertilization as a technology that serves life. In the end, even Catholics may begin to realize that their Church's teaching against all laboratory production of human life contained a great deal of wisdom after all.

Notes

1. "Protection of Human Subjects: Fetuses, Pregnant Women, and In Vitro Fertilization," 40 *Fed. Reg.* 33525-52 (August 8, 1975) at 33529.
2. "Report of the Ethics Advisory Board," 44 *Federal Register* 35033-58 (June 18, 1979) at 35055, 35057.
3. Section 121(c) of the NIH Revitalization Act of 1993, Public Law 103-43, rescinding 45 CFR §46.204(d).
4. National Institutes of Health, Transcript, Human Embryo Research Panel, February 3, 1994, pp. 97-8 (statement by panel chairman Steven Muller).
5. See National Institutes of Health, *Report of the Human Embryo Research Panel* (1994).
6. Editorial, "Embryos: Drawing the Line," *The Washington Post*, October 2, 1994, p. C6.
7. Editorial, "Embryo Research Is Inhuman," *Chicago Sun-Times*, October 10, 1994, p. 25.
8. The current version of this law is Section 510 of the Departments of Labor, Health and Human Services, and Education, and Related Agencies Appropriations Act for Fiscal Year 2002, Public Law 107-116.
9. See National Institutes of Health, Transcript, 69th Meeting of the Advisory Committee to the Director, December 1, 1994: pp. 114 (Dr. Snyderman on acclimating the public to research on "spare" embryos before taking the further step of specially creating embryos for research); 134-5 (Dr. Trojanowski on pressing forward with the development of embryonic cell lines first to win public support for embryo research); 139-140 (Dr. Corlin on persuading key members of Congress that such research may help members of their own families with certain illnesses).
10. Hearing on Stem Cell Research before the U.S. Senate Appropriations Subcommittee on Labor, Health and Human Services, Education and Related Agencies, December 2, 1998.
11. "Report of the Ethics Advisory Board," note 2 supra, at 35056 (the early human embryo deserves "profound respect" as a form of developing human life); *Report of the Human Embryo Research Panel*, note 5 supra, p. 2 ("the preimplantation human embryo warrants serious moral consideration as a developing form of human life."); National Bioethics Advisory Commission, *Ethical Issues in Human Stem Cell Research* (September 1999), Vol. I, pp. ii, 2 (citing broad agreement in our society that "human embryos deserve respect as a form of human life").
12. See 45 CFR §§ 46.208(a) (fetus protected as human subject from research risks), 46.203(c) ("fetus" includes the product of conception from implantation onward).
13. See Secretariat for Pro-Life Activities, U.S. Conference of Catholic Bishops, "Fact Sheet: The NIH Proposal for Stem Cell Research Is a Crime," www.usccb.org/prolife/issues/bioethic/states701.htm.

14. See: U.S. Conference of Catholic Bishops press release, "New Poll: Americans Oppose Destructive Embryo Research, Support Alternatives," June 8, 2001, www.usccb.org/comm/archives/2001/01-101.htm; Id., "Americans Overwhelmingly Oppose Human Cloning," June 7, 2001, www.usccb.org/comm/archives/2001/01-098.htm; Stop Human Cloning press release, "New Poll: American People Oppose All Human Cloning, Support President Bush's Call for a Comprehensive Ban," April 22, 2002, www.cloninginformation.org/prps/shc_02-04-22.htm.

15. *Ethical Issues in Human Stem Cell Research*, note 11 supra, p. 53.

16. See Testimony of Richard M. Doerflinger before the Subcommittee on Labor, Health and Human Services, and Education, Senate Appropriations Committee, July 18, 2001, www.usccb.org/prolife/issues/bioethic/stemcelltest71801.htm.

17. According to bioethicist Glenn McGee, a supporter of embryonic stem cell research: "The emerging truth in the lab is that pluripotent stem cells are hard to rein in. The potential that they would explode into a cancerous mass after a stem cell transplant might turn out to be the Pandora's box of stem cell research." See E. Jonietz, "Innovation: Sourcing Stem Cells," *Technology Review*, January/February 2001, p. 32.

18. "Human Cloning Prohibition Act of 2001," in *Congressional Record*, July 31, 2001, pp. H4916-45 (recorded vote at p. H4945).

19. White House press release, "Radio Address by the President to the Nation," August 11, 2001, www.whitehouse.gov/news/releases/2001/08/20010811-1.html.

20. "The logic of the American free enterprise system suggests that President Bush's decision is going to provide incentive for the private sector to get more involved. And once the basic research is conducted, the private sector likely will have great incentive to step in and transform this basic research into therapies for disease." Testimony of HHS Secretary Tommy Thompson before the Senate Health, Education, Labor and Pensions Committee, Sept. 5, 2001, www.hhs.gov/news/speech/2001/010905.html.

21. J. Cibelli et al., "Rapid Communication: Somatic Cell Nuclear Transfer in Humans: Pronuclear and Early Embryonic Development," in 2 *e-biomed: The Journal of Regenerative Medicine* 25 (Nov. 26, 2001), accessible at www.liebertpub.com/ebi/default1.asp.

22. S. 1899, Human Cloning Prohibition Act of 2001, introduced by Sen. Sam Brownback et al. on January 28, 2002.

23. See: S. 1758, Human Cloning Prohibition Act of 2001, introduced by Sen. Dianne Feinstein et al. on December 3, 2001; S. 1893, Human Cloning Ban and Stem Cell Research Protection Act of 2002, introduced by Sen. Tom Harkin et al. on January 24, 2002; S. 2439, Human Cloning Prohibition Act of 2002, introduced by Sen. Arlen Specter et al. on May 1, 2002.

24. See Gail Quinn, Executive Director, USCCB Secretariat for Pro-Life Activities, Letter to Senate on the Harkin/Feinstein Cloning Bill (S. 2439), May 20, 2002, www.usccb.org/prolife/issues/bioethic/clonelet52002.htm.

25. See Statement by Daniel J. Bryant, Assistant Attorney General, Office of Leg-

islative Affairs, U.S. Department of Justice to the House Government Reform Committee, May 15, 2002, at www.cloninginformation.org/congressional_ testimony/bryant_02-05-15.htm.

26. See Secretariat for Pro-Life Activities, U.S. Conference of Catholic Bishops, "Fact Sheet: What is Human Cloning?," www.usccb.org/prolife/issues/bioethic/ clonfact202.htm.

27. See N. Munro, "The New Patent Puzzle," in *National Journal*, March 2, 2002, pp. 628-9.

28. S. 2076, introduced by Sen. Byron Dorgan on April 9, 2002. After public outcry arose over this language and his co-sponsors rescinded their support, Senator Dorgan obtained the Senate's consent to change the language while retaining this bill number (see *Congressional Record*, June 10, 2002, p. S5317).

29. See: New Scientist news service, "Therapeutic cloning 'proof of principle'," 2 June 2002, www.newscientist.com/news/news.jsp?id=ns99992356; Americans to Ban Cloning, "Why the 'Successful' Mouse 'Therapeutic' Cloning Really Didn't Work," www.cloninginformation.org/info/unsuccessful_mouse_ therapy.htm.

30. In the words of Ian Wilmut, creator of "Dolly" the sheep: "Cloning of the kind that we have developed at Roslin and PPL makes it possible in principle to apply all the immense power of genetic engineering and genomics to animals... and human beings, of course, are animals too." I. Wilmut et al., *The Second Creation* (Farrar Straus and Giroux 2000), p. 9.

31. See J. Mendible, "Genetically Designed Pets to Fit the Owner's Taste," at Suite101.com, July 13, 2001 (www.suite101.com/article.cfm/4866/74458).

32. L. Silver, *Remaking Eden: Cloning and Beyond in a Brave New World* (New York: Avon Books 1997), pp. 281-93.

CHAPTER 9

The Constitutionality of Recent Pro-life Legislation

Gerard V. Bradley

My subject is proposed federal legislation, not enacted laws. I aim, more specifically, to look at the constitutional issues surrounding three pending pro-life bills. They are, in the order I shall discuss them: The Unborn Victims of Violence Act, which would ban feticide; The Born Alive Infants Protection Act,[1] which would ban infanticide; and The Human Cloning Prohibition Act, which would ban all human cloning.

Three preliminary comments: One is that each of these federal bills corresponds to either pending legislation or to enacted laws in many states. I do not explore those state counterparts. Another preliminary observation is that, as I compose these comments, each of the three bills awaits action in the United States Senate. Each has already received House approval, and President Bush says he will sign any of the bills, which pass both houses of Congress. Finally, I confine my discussion to constitutional questions concerning the protection of nascent life. Given the Constitution's broad phrasing, and the expansive manner of its recent judicial interpretation, this focus does not exclude all moral philosophical considerations. Still, the task I set for myself is to examine the constitutionality of each insofar as these are pro-life bills. Wider considerations are brought into view only as constitutional concerns require. And I leave aside another kind of constitutional issue, one the lawyers call "jurisdiction." Let me explain.

Our national government possesses extensive but not indefinite powers, large but not unlimited jurisdiction. Ours is a national government of specific and enumerated powers. It possesses no general power to protect persons, including unborn persons, against private violence. The closest the national government comes to such an authority is the power conferred upon Congress to "enforce" the Fourteenth Amendment's guarantee to all "persons" of the "equal protection" of state laws, including state laws against physical harm. Upon an appropriate finding of fact by Congress that some identifiable class of persons—say, a racial or ethnic minority, or a particularly vulnerable and politically powerless group, like the infirm or unborn—is unequally exposed to private violence by lax enforcement of state homicide laws, direct federal protection against such discrimination would be constitutionally required. This would be a kind of federal back-up, or safety net, for the protection of life. Protecting life in the first instance, on the front lines, would still principally be a state duty.

What this all means is that each and every piece of federal legislation, including the three I examine here, must be an exercise of some *specific* power allocated by our Constitution to Congress. Examples of these powers include that over interstate commerce and with regard to all military activities. Elaborate case law has grown up to define the reach, or scope, of these powers, especially the commerce power. What I leave aside, then, is consideration of how each of these three proposals fits within the defined framework of federal power. All I choose to say here is that all three bills *do* fit within current definitions of congressional power.

The Unborn Victims of Violence Act

This proposed bill—designated S. 1673—makes certain instances of feticide federal crimes. Essentially, the proposal says that whoever assaults a pregnant woman, where that assault would already be a federal offense, commits a *separate* offense if that woman's unborn child is harmed, or killed. An example of a federally cognizable assault would be an attack upon a servicewoman.

Nothing in the Act affects, much less unconstitutionally restricts, the woman's right to terminate her pregnancy. One section of the Act makes this allowance for the effect of *Roe v. Wade* unmistakably clear. No woman may be prosecuted under this Act "with respect to her unborn child." No woman engaged in predicate criminal conduct may be prosecuted for harm to her child, even where she did not intend to abort. So, a woman engaged in a hijacking or assault upon a federal juror or in animal terrorism or in *any* covered activity and who, as a result (of flight or some mishap) causes harm or death to her *own* fetus, is beyond prosecution under this Act, even though she may be liable for hijacking or assault upon a juror or animal terrorism. The Act simply does not inhibit the woman's freedom to choose whether to bear a child or not.

In fact, one of the state interests, which might be said to be promoted by the Act, is precisely the liberty articulated in *Roe*. A woman's freedom to carry a baby to term is inhibited or denied by conduct that results in harm or death to her unborn child.

Someone might object that the Act, in its protection of what the Act calls "unborn children," is somehow inconsistent with *Roe v. Wade*. Is there no difference, the objection might hold, between this Act and a flat congressional declaration that the unborn *are* persons? And is not that declaration inconsistent with *Roe*, and the cases following it?

The answer to this challenge would very likely have to be yes if the Supreme Court in *Roe,* or in some other case, held that the unborn are *not* persons. But the Court has never so held. The *Roe* court said that it did not "need [to] resolve the difficult question of when life begins."[2] The Court there said the "the judiciary…is not in a position to speculate as to the answer."[1] In no general or broad way, moreover, did the Court hold that the states or the Congress operated under a similar disability. All that the Court held in this regard was that Texas (and thus any other governmental body, including for argument sake, the Congress) "could not override the rights of the pregnant woman" by adopting an answer to the question of when life begins, that she could not be deprived of all freedom of choice by the consequences of legislation regarding the beginning of life.[3]

This Act does not affect, much less "override," the rights of any pregnant woman. The *Roe* court opined that the unborn were not to be considered persons in the "whole" sense, an opinion consistent with treating the unborn as persons for some purposes, like inheritance and tort injury, purposes which the *Roe* court itself recognized as legitimate.

This understanding of *Roe* was explicitly confirmed by the Supreme Court in the 1989 *Webster* decision. There the state of Missouri had legislated that the "life of each human being begins at conception," and the "unborn children have protectable interests in life, health, and well being."[4] The 8th Circuit Court of Appeals seems to have adopted the view of *Roe* stated as an "objection" here, that the state had, in light of *Roe*, "impermissibly" adopted a "theory of when life begins."[5] But, the Supreme Court reversed this part of the 8th Circuit holding, stating that its own prior decisions, including *Roe,* meant "only that a state could not justify an abortion regulation *otherwise invalid under Roe v. Wade* on the ground that it embodied the state's view."[6] Since this Act in no way is questionable under *Roe* apart from the viewpoint issue, the matter is settled: Congress is as free as was the state of Missouri to conclude and to enforce outside the parameters of *Roe,* its view that life begins at conception. If there remains something anomalous about the situation, it is an anomaly engendered by *Roe*, and not by this Act.

The Born-Alive Infants Protection Act

This bill—denominated H.R. 4292—is exclusively a definitional provision, identical in structure and function to the provision of the United States Code, which it would, if enacted, follow. That preceding section, which happens to be the Defense of Marriage Act, defines "marriage" and "spouse" for the purpose of construing "any Act of Congress, or of any ruling, regulation, or interpretation of the various administrative bureaus of the United States." This Act defines the words "person," "human being," "child," and "individual" for identical purposes, as including (practically speaking) every baby who has emerged entirely from the womb, alive.

Someone might object that the Act, in its definition of "person" or "child," is somehow inconsistent with *Roe* and cases following it. At least as used in assault or homicide statutes to protect an infant born after a failed abortion, someone might object that this legislative definition abridges a woman's freedom to abort. Is there not, at least, a broad spirit of *Roe* which might limit application of the Act? What of the limit case of a woman who exercises her liberty to terminate a pregnancy—who thus wishes to avoid maternity—but who ends up the mother of an infant anyway? Is there, at least in this situation, a violation of the spirit of *Roe*, if Congress can "force" her to be a mother against her will?

There is language in the *Roe* opinion to support this objection. The *Roe* Court catalogued the "detriment" the government would "impose" upon a pregnant woman by denying her the freedom to choose an abortion:

> Maternity, or additional offspring, may force upon the woman a distressful life and future. Psychological harm may be imminent. Mental and physical health may be taxed by childcare. There is also the distress, for all concerned, associated with the unwanted child, and there is the problem

of bringing a child into a family already unable, psychologically and otherwise, to care for it. In other cases, as in this one, the additional difficulties and continuing stigma of unwed motherhood may be involved.[7]

Quite obviously these are "detriments" not of pregnancy, but of having and raising a child. Thus, is there not some very brief time *after* live birth for the woman to decide whether to keep the baby?

The answer as a matter of constitutional law is surely not. The obviously post-natal nature of the "detriments" "imposed" upon the pregnant woman denied access to abortion supports, rather than undermines, this conclusion. Beginning with *Roe* itself, the Supreme Court has consistently, and unanimously as far as I can tell, drawn the line of a woman's authority to control the consequences of her reproductive activity at live birth, the precise line followed by the Act.

In its first favorable reference ever to abortion the Supreme Court spoke in a 1971 case of a protected choice to "bear" or "beget" a child. "Bear," in the common understanding, means "to give birth." It has no post-natal reference; when birth is concluded, a child has been born. *Roe v. Wade* consistently, without exception, referred to abortion as the "termination of pregnancy." Nowhere did the *Roe* Court even hint that "abortion" might refer to the termination of a born child. The *Roe* Court often referred to "potential life," and used that term interchangeably with the "fetus," or the child *in utero*. All these terms were contrasted to the child born alive. The phrase "live birth" appears many times as the analytical divide in the *Roe* opinion, indicating in every case that no one on the Court questioned the appropriateness of legal protection of the just-born infant. Most important, in its discussion of what counts as a "person" within the meaning of the Constitution, the *Roe* Court again drew the line at birth. After listing the many uses of "person" in the Constitution, the Court concluded that it applied only "post-natally." At the same time, the abortion liberty extended only pre-natally.

In truth, the most plausible interpretation of *Roe,* as it bears upon this Act, is not that Congress has violated or even stretched the Constitution. On the most plausible interpretation of *Roe*, Congress has codified a constitutional command.

The born-alive rule is, moreover, essential to making any sense of the *Roe* Court's term "potential life." The *Roe* Court said that "viable" fetuses were those capable of living outside the womb, independent of the mother. These unborn children the Court nevertheless referred to as possessing, or being, "potential life," which the state might protect even by proscribing abortions (save for those necessary to the life or health of the mother). But, what is "potential" about these "lives"? Already (actually) able to live outside the womb, the "potentiality" could, it seems, only be spatial: able now to live (to be "life"), but only "potentially" outside the womb. Simply put, "potential life" refers to the same analytical divide we find in the Act: "potential" persons become *actual* persons precisely by being born.

The Court's line drawing was supported by the spirit of its ruling, which was only one part animated by a woman's liberty. The Court stressed in unmistakably clear terms that this liberty was not absolute, and that it was limited by the social interest in protecting "potential life"—a child in *utero*—and, after birth, by the exceptionless protection of new persons.

Finally, I turn to a more modest objection, one based upon the Supreme Court's decision in the summer of 2000, striking down laws that made partial-birth abortion illegal. The objection is this: might not this Act interfere with some abortions, especially those occurring in late term? Does "complete expulsion or extraction" from the mother—the earmark of live birth, under this Act—clearly delineate, and protect, *all* "abortions"? Might some "abortions," at least according to medical authorities, be prohibited—or chilled—by the Act's protection of born-alive infants?

Again, the answer is, no. According to the very same authorities depended upon by the Court in its decision in favor of partial-birth abortion, the Act's definition of "born alive" as "complete expulsion or extraction" accurately describes "birth" which, according to the same authorities, terminates a "pregnancy." *Webster's Third Edition* defines "birth" as "the act of coming forth from the womb," "the emergence of a new individual from the body of its parent."[8] "Pregnant" is defined as "containing unborn young within the body," "preparing to bring forth" an unborn individual. [7] *Maloy's Medical Dictionary for Lawyers* defines pregnancy as "the state of being with young; preparing to bring forth" [9]; "birth" is "the act of coming into life, or being born."[10] The *Oxford-English Dictionary* (2nd edition) defines "birth" as "the bearing of offspring"; "bringing forth." "Pregnant," according to the OED, is "with child or young."

Abortion, these sources and the cases make clear, refers exclusively to terminating a "pregnancy." Another way to terminate a "pregnancy," it is equally clear, is to give "birth." Having given "birth" by completely expelling the child from the womb, the Act assures equal protection of the law to the person just born. The woman is not then prohibited, by this or any other act, from securing or completing an "abortion." From the moment of birth on, "abortion" is, according to standard medical usage, impossible. No "pregnancy" remains to be terminated.

The Human Cloning Prohibition Act

Several putatively anti-cloning bills have been introduced in Congress over the last couple years. The main difference between the two classes of putative bans is this: some "bans" would outlaw only what is usually called "reproductive" cloning, the attempt to impregnate a woman with a cloned embryo, with the hope of bringing to live birth the genetic replica of someone else. These "bans" would allow for so-called "therapeutic" cloning. This endeavor involves creating human embryos, in order to experiment upon them, and thereby to destroy them.

The better bills ban *all* cloning whatsoever. I consider objections to such comprehensive bans, starting with the claim that Supreme Court precedent gives persons a right of privacy broad enough to include the choice to reproduce by cloning.

This objection overstates what the Court has decided. According to the Supreme Court, its privacy cases have established constitutional protection for the right: to marry; to have children; to direct the education and upbringing of one's children; to marital privacy; to use contraception; to bodily integrity; and to abortion. Only two of these rights are in the neighborhood of cloning. For the proposition in favor of a right to "have children," the Court relied upon a 1942 decision against involuntary sterilization. For the right to "marital privacy" the Court cited *Griswold,* its 1965 decision in favor a right of married couples to use contraception. There is therefore no Supreme Court authority nearly in line against a ban on human cloning.

There is, generally, Supreme Court precedent in favor of a woman's right to decide, by herself, whether to "bear or beget" a child. But the cases giving rise to that right make clear that "begotten" is surely not made—or cloned. And "bear" unequivocally refers to the abortion liberty. There is also authority for the proposition that, in no exact sense, one has a right not to become a parent against one's wishes. But that right is limited to pregnant women; a man either deceived or the victim of contraceptive failure has no constitutional traction whatsoever upon the decision of the woman to abort their child, or to carry their child to term. Besides, this woman's right is surely asymmetrical. A right *not* to be a parent does not imply or entail a right, simply, to *be* a parent.

No case, *in any court,* has ever held in favor of a constitutional right to reproduction by cloning. In fact, no case has ever held that anyone has a right to reproduce by *in vitro fertilization* (IVF).

To generate a "privacy" argument against a comprehensive cloning ban and in favor of reproductive cloning, one would have to go beyond *all* prior holdings of *all* the courts. The only way that I can think of to make that argument would detach a commodious phrase, such as the "right to have children," from its jurisprudential moorings, and then (somehow) maintain that the broad concept implies a right to reproduce by cloning. But no such argument could possibly succeed, as I understand the Supreme Court's stance towards all such novel claims of constitutional rights.

The Court has repeatedly emphasized two fundamental requirements for any "privacy" argument in favor of an unrecognized liberty interest. First, the asserted liberty must be, objectively speaking, "deeply rooted in this nation's history and tradition." Cloning clearly does not satisfy this requirement. Not only is it an entirely new technology. By reducing reproduction to asexual replication, it is radically unlike all rights sounding in "reproductive liberty" heretofore recognized. In other words, even argument by analogy will not work for cloning.

Second, the Supreme Court has cautioned, in very strong terms, against arguments relying upon spacious phrasing. The Court has *insisted* that the asserted liberty be described in specific, concrete terms. Vague, open-ended generalities will not do.

According to this second requirement, no general "right to reproduce," "to be a parent," or "to have a child" will be credited, either as a conclusion or as a premise, in any argument in the Supreme Court. The Court will insist that a claimant defend a right *specifically* to cloning. Given the high burden of persuasion imposed by the high Court upon such claimants, the chances of success are virtually nil.

The Supreme Court has said: "We must therefore 'exercise the utmost care whenever we are asked to break new ground in this field'...lest the liberty protected by the Due Process Clause be subtly transformed into the policy preferences of the members of this Court."[11] This statement of judicial restraint implies that "policy" is the business of Congress, at least where the Court does not stake a claim to constitutional supervision. The Court has not and, in my judgment, will not, with regard to cloning.

Let me explain, in one more way, why members of Congress are constrained in this matter by their sworn duty to uphold the Constitution and to legislate for the common good, *unconstrained* by judicial doctrine. It is true that cloning has *some* features in common with acts that are constitutionally protected. Cloning is, for example, a way to have a baby, and people (women especially) have a right to decide whether to have a baby. Also, let us say for argument sake, that individuals have a right to have babies outside of marriage. (They do, in the limited sense of being immune to criminal, and practically all civil, penalties for doing so. But individuals do not actually have a constitutional right to unwed parenthood.) Again, you do not have to be married to have a baby by cloning.

But, to observe that cloning is *like* protected acts in *two* respects is not saying much. It is not saying much because cloning posses *several additional* features, and it is precisely those *additional features* which are the grounds of the proposed ban—features included in the description of cloning as the asexual manufacture of genetic replicas. We may presume that members of Congress voting for this bill do not do so because they are opposed to people having babies, even outside of wedlock. So far considered, then, members do not adopt as a reason for action any adverse moral judgment upon any act (or feature of an act) declared by courts to be private, or none of Congress's business. Congress, in this thought experiment, regulates *only* for reasons entirely left open to their policy judgment by the courts. There is no good reason to anticipate authoritative judicial action, which would block congressional action upon those reasons. There is every good reason to conclude that none will be forthcoming.

A comparison might help to make this point clearer. There is no doubt now that movies are a constitutionally protected mode of speech. Individuals therefore may be said to have a right to make movies. And, so long as amenities are preserved, they have a right to make movies about children, using child actors. Francis Ford Coppola, for example, may be said to have a right to do a remake of "Heidi," using the Olson twins as stars. Should Congress attempt to suppress this project, so far described, Congress would have acted unconstitutionally. But, does anyone think that if a particular director wished to make a *porno* version of "Heidi," using child actresses, he has a *right* to do so? That Congress would be acting *unconstitutionally* by prohibiting child pornography?

Of course not, even though porno "Heidi" possesses, we may suppose, every feature of Coppola's "Heidi." And that is because porno "Heidi" possesses *one* additional feature—sexual exploitation of children—which is not constitutionally protected. Cloning possesses *many* unprotected features.

A Note on IVF

As I noted above, no court in any American jurisdiction has held in favor of a federal constitutional right to have a child by *in vitro fertilization*. It is nevertheless permitted in most, if not all, jurisdictions. Does approval of

IVF imply or suggest approval of cloning? Is a ban on cloning somehow inconsistent with approval of IVF? Would a projected court decision in favor of a constitutional right to IVF implicitly undermine the constitutionality of this bill? The answer to all these questions is "No."

IVF and cloning are both methods of asexual human reproduction, which rely upon scientific technique to bring an embryo into being. Both techniques require the implantation of the embryo into a woman's womb in order to bring forth a fully developed baby approximately nine months later. But, otherwise, cloning is radically discontinuous with IVF, and much more distant from human reproduction as traditionally morally approved, and as recognized in Due Process cases.

For the principle of reproduction in IVF procedures is the human couple. The child born is the issue of two parents, who become mother and father of that child. That child is genetically unique, the unrepeatable combination (genetically speaking) of his/her mom and dad. None of the cloning problems of individuality and identity plague IVF. Though assisted by the lab technician, the embryo is created in IVF as it is within the woman's body in intercourse: by the spontaneous fusion of gametes—egg and sperm. Most important, because of the unique and spontaneous genetic constitution of the IVF baby, there is scarcely a trace of the manufactured product status that would be characteristic of cloning.

By contrast, cloning is the impersonal, individualized undertaking to make a person to the specifications of a single (genetic) parent. It is replication, not true reproduction, and it is radically de-humanized. The way to think of IVF in relation to cloning is an aggravated form of the relation between the two Heidi movies, as I described the hypothetical above.

Notes

1. In August of 2002, President Bush signed into law the Born Alive Infants Protection Act.
2. *Roe v Wade*, 410 U.S. 159 (1973).
3. Ibid., 410 U.S. 162
4. *Webster v Reproductive Health Services*, 492 U.S. 504 (1989).
5. Ibid., 492 U.S. 505
6. Ibid., 492 U.S. 506 (emphasis added)
7. *Roe v. Wade*, 410 U.S. 153 (1973).

8. *Webster's Third Edition*, 221
9. *Maloy's Medical Dictionary for Lawyers (3rd. 1960); 581*
10. *Maloy's Medical Dictionary for Lawyers (3rd. 1960); 104*
11. *Washington v. Glucksberg*, 521 U.S. 702 (1997).

CONTRIBUTORS

Steven Bozza, MA is Director of Family Ministries for the Diocese of Camden New Jersey. He also is an Adjunct Professor of Biomedical Ethics at Our Lady of Lourdes Medical Center School of Nursing and Adjunct Professor of Moral Theology at Immaculata College in Pennsylvania. He holds a Master of Arts degree in Moral Theology from St. Charles Seminary and is the author of several books including *Begotten Not Made: a Guide for the Pastoral Care of Couples Experiencing Infertility* and *Christian Married Life.* He lives with his wife of 16 years, Janice, in Collingswood New Jersey and has one step son.

Gerard Bradley, J.D. is Professor of Law at the University of Notre Dame, where he has taught since 1992. During the Fall of 2001, he was Visiting Professor of Law at Ave Maria School of Law in Ann Arbor, Michigan. He taught at the University of Illinois College of Law from 1983 until 1992. Professor Bradley has published widely in the fields of constitutional law, legal philosophy, and on subjects at the intersection of law and morality. He has testified before Congressional committees on many occasions, including testimony on cloning and abortion-related issues. From 1995 until 2001 Professor Bradley served as President of the Fellowship of Catholic Scholars.

Richard M. Doerflinger, PhD is Deputy Director of the Secretariat for Pro-Life Activities, United States Conference of Catholic Bishops, where he has worked for 21 years. Among his duties is the preparation of policy statements and congressional testimony on abortion, euthanasia, embryo research, human cloning, and other medical-moral issues for the bishops' conference. He holds a M.A. in Divinity from the University of Chicago and is Adjunct Fellow in Bioethics and Public Policy at the National Catholic Bioethics Center in Boston. He has published widely on this and other medical-moral issues, including contributions to *Hastings Center Report, Duquesne Law Review, the Kennedy Institute of Ethics Journal, the Encyclopedia of Catholic Doctrine published by Our Sunday Visitor Press, the National Catholic Bioethics Quarterly*, and the *American Journal of Bioethics*.

Jean Bethke Elshtain, PhD is the Laura Spelman Rockefeller Professor of Social and Political Ethics at the University of Chicago. She is the author or editor of many books including: *Public Man, Private Woman: Woman in Social and Political Thought, Meditations on Modern Political Thought, and Democracy on Trial, Politics and the Human Body* and *Just War Theory*. Dr. Elshtain is also the author of over four hundred articles and essays in scholarly journals and journals of civic opinion. In 1996, she was elected a Fellow of the American Academy of Arts and Sciences. She is the recipient of seven honorary degrees and co-director of the recently established Pew Forum on Religion and American Public Life.

Francis Cardinal George, O.M.I. is the archbishop of the city of Chicago. He entered the Missionary Oblates of Mary Immaculate in 1957 and was ordained a priest on December 21, 1963. Cardinal George has served as Bishop in the diocese of Yakima and as Archbishop in the city of Portland. He was installed as Archbishop of Chicago on May 27, 1996 and named Cardinal by Pope John Paul II January 18, 1998.

Patrick Guinan, M.D. is the clinical associate professor in the Department of Urology at the University of Illinois at Chicago College of Medicine. He is president of the Catholic Physician's Guild of Chicago. Dr. Guinan received his B.S. from Marquette University in 1958 and his M.D. from Marquette School of Medicine in 1962. He subsequently received a Masters degree in Public Health from Columbia University in 1965 and a Masters degree in Surgery from the University of Illinois in 1983. Dr. Guinan has published two books entitled *Core Readings in Catholic Medical Ethics* and *Genetics: a Catholic Perspective* as well as over 200 scientific publications.

John M. Hass, PhD, STL, M Div. is the President of the National Catholic Bioethics Center in Boston, MA. The Center was established in 1972 to investigate research problems in medical ethics and to apply the teachings of the Catholic Church to specific medical issues emerging from advances in medicine, the life sciences, and civil law. Dr. Haas received his PhD in Moral Theology from the Catholic University of America and his STL in Moral Theology from the University of Fribourg, Switzerland. He has served as a member of the Medical Moral Commission of the Archdiocese of Philadelphia and testified before the Massachusetts Legislature, the US Senate Committee on Health and Public Safety and the President's National Bioethics Advisory Commission. Author, editor, lecturer and father of nine children are among his invaluable roles.

Patrick Lee, PhD is professor of philosophy at the Franciscan University of Steubenville. He grew up in Dallas Texas, received his B.A. from the University of Dallas in 1974, his M.A. in philosophy from Niagara University in 1977, and his Ph. D. in philosophy from Marquette University in 1980. He is a specialist in ethics and in the philosophy of St. Thomas Aquinas. He has published articles in various scholarly journals, such as *American Catholic Philosophical Quarterly, International Philosophical Quarterly*, and *Faith and Philosophy*. His book, *Abortion and Unborn Human Life,* appeared in 1996, and is available from Catholic University of America Press, or from Amazon.com. He is now working on a book together with Robert P. George, tentatively titled, "Dualism and Contemporary Ethical Issues." He and his wife Rita have nine children (ages 5 to 29) and four grandchildren (from 4 mo. in utero to 5).

William E. May, PhD is Michael J. McGivney Professor of Moral Theology at the John Paul Institute for Studies on Marriage and Family, where he has taught since 1991 after completing 20 years of teaching at The Catholic University of America. He is the author of several books, including *Catholic Bioethics and the Gift of Human Life, An Introduction to Moral Theology, Marriage: The Rock on Which the Family Is Built* and over 200 articles in scholarly and professional journals. He is a consultant to the National Catholic Center for Bioethics and from 1986-1996 was appointed by John Paul II to serve on the International Theological Commission. Professor May has been married to Patricia Ann Keck for 43 years. They are the grandparents of 10, with more, God willing, to come.

Daniel P. Toma, PhD received his Ph.D. in Biology from the University of Illinois, Urbana-Champaign in 1999. His thesis work involved the molecular genetic basis of behavioral development in honeybees. He is presently doing post-doctoral research in the lab of Dr. Ralph Greenspan at the Neurosciences Institute in San Diego, CA. His work there involves the mechanisms of gene interaction in the brain controlling responses to gravity in the fruit fly. He is a life long student of philosophy and theology and is currently working on several publications discussing the relationship of science, philosophy, and theology.

INDEX